RACHEL HILLER is a clinical research psychologist in developmental psychopathology at the University of Bath, UK. She worked for a number of years at the Child & Adolescent Sleep Clinic in South Australia, where she specialised in CBT treatments for childhood sleep disorders. Her work in the UK continues to focus on helping families of children with anxiety-based disorders.

MICHAEL GRADISAR is a clinical psychologist and professor in clinical child psychology at Flinders University, Australia. He is also the director of the Child & Adolescent Sleep Clinic, where he has helped hundreds of school-aged children (and their parents) to sleep better through the night.

HELPING YOUR CHILD WITH SLEEP PROBLEMS

A Self-Help Guide for Parents

Rachel Hiller and Michael Gradisar

ROBINSON

ROBINSON

First published in Great Britain in 2018 by Robinson

Copyright © Rachel Hiller and Michael Gradisar, 2018

1 3 5 7 9 10 8 6 4 2

A CIP catalogue record for this book is available from the British
Library

ISBN: 978-1-47213-872-9

Designed and typeset by Initial Typesetting Services, Edinburgh
Printed and bound in Great Britain by CPI Group (UK),
Croydon CR0 4YY

Papers used by Robinson are from well-managed forests and other
responsible sources

www.littlebrown.co.uk

Contents

PART III

Preface

At some point in their development, many children will experience trouble sleeping. The delay tactics come out – they are thirsty, they need the toilet, they are not tired . . . the list goes on. Perhaps they have a big test at school or have heard a story in the playground that made them feel worried and they have a few nights where they are more resistant about going to bed than usual. This can be a normal part of childhood. However, in some cases, sleep problems can last for many months, or even years, and night-time can become a time of high stress, anxiety and many tears (from the parent and child!). We know that many parents feel uncertain about the best way to support their child's sleep problems or night-time anxiety.

Is my child's sleep normal? Is it abnormal? Should I ignore them? Should I stay with them? Will they grow out of it?

Coupled with this stress, sleep seems to be an area where *everyone* has an opinion on what you should do, or what you are doing 'wrong'. Wading through these opinions can be a further source of stress for many parents.

Books on sleep are available in abundance. However, if you look in your local bookstore or online you will see that most books target infant sleep or adult sleep (e.g. insomnia). There is very little information about how to help your older child sleep. This is problematic, as we know that approximately half of all children will experience sleep problems at some point. We also know, from our clinical work, that many parents spend months or years trying to work out the best way to help their child sleep and – amongst the various opinions and strategies provided by well-meaning people – parents can find it very difficult to work out what the best techniques are to help their child sleep. We would like parents to be able to have access to a resource where they can learn techniques to improve their child's sleep, based on the best scientific information that is currently available. Therefore, through this book, we have provided parents with step-by-step information about how to help their child overcome their sleep problem. This book is aimed at children aged 5 to 12 years old, but you may see similar patterns of sleep in your slightly younger or older children who could also benefit from these strategies.

So who are we?

We are both clinical psychologists who specialise in working with children, adolescents and their families. For the past sixteen years, Michael has worked with children, teenagers and adults with sleep problems. In 2005 he opened the Child & Adolescent Sleep Clinic at Flinders University in South Australia, where he has pioneered the development of cognitive and behavioural treatments for childhood sleep disorders. In 2011, Rachel joined this clinic, where she specialised in cognitive and behavioural treatments for children and teens with sleep problems, before relocating to the UK to continue her research and clinical work in the area of clinical child psychology.

Through our clinical work and research, we have seen hundreds of children and families who are struggling with sleep problems. While every family we saw was unique, we continued to see many similarities in the stories we heard from parents. In particular, many parents were very unsure about the best way to respond to their child's sleep problems, particularly when it stemmed from anxiety. By the time they had come to us at the clinic, many had been dealing with their child's sleep problem for years – sometimes over a decade. Maybe for many years it had been manageable. They might have sat with their child while they fell asleep, but it only took 15 minutes. Their child may have slept in the parents'/parent's bed, but this was okay for a while. Often, as they reached school age (e.g. around 4–5 years old) the sleep problems became more difficult to manage. They completely ruled the family's evenings. Parents hadn't had their bed to themselves for years, or hadn't had any time for themselves in the evening. They themselves might be sleep deprived from being woken during the night. Of course, overwhelmingly, they were worried about their child being very anxious, but also what it might mean if their child is sleep deprived. Their child might be too anxious to go to school camps or trips or to sleepovers with friends, or even to stay with their relatives. In some cases, their child might be able to do all of these things, but when they were at home with Mum or Dad they found it very difficult to fall asleep – causing lots of stress and anxiety for everyone involved.

In this book we cover a range of sleep problems that we most commonly see in our clinical work. This includes children who find it very difficult to sleep without a parent present, or where they are very anxious at night-time. We also discuss parasomnias (i.e. when your child performs a behaviour while they are 'asleep'), including bed-wetting, sleep-walking and night terrors. The approaches we discuss are the same approaches that we use in our clinical work, and the examples we provide are based on different families that we have seen over the years (with names changed). Treatments are based on cognitive and behavioural approaches. These approaches were originally designed for the treatment of adults with insomnia and over the years have been adapted for use with children. Importantly, these treatments have also undergone testing via research studies, where we, and other researchers, have shown that they can be highly effective in combating child sleep problems. Cognitive and behavioural strategies to target sleep problems are the 'gold standard' method (that is, the techniques recommended by experts on the basis of the current evidence) of improving childhood sleep problems, particularly when they are related to anxiety.

But before we begin – we know that many parents feel a lot of guilt around their child's sleep, especially when their child is very anxious at night. No parent likes to see their child anxious or distressed. In our clinical work, parents often ask us questions such as:

Have I caused it? Am I making it worse?

Sometimes even well-meaning advice from a relative or friend can make a parent feel as if they have somehow failed. Nevertheless, it is important to note that there are many different factors that can cause a sleep problem to develop, some of which we will discuss in Part I of this book. Sleep problems are rarely caused by one single issue. However, parents do hold the key to helping their child overcome their sleep problem. The aim of this book is to help equip parents and children with the skills to face the child's worries during the night, and to restore better sleep practices. This is partly through identifying and shifting bedtime practices that may have been used to reduce anxiety in the short term, but may have unknowingly contributed to the maintenance of longer-term sleep problems. Ultimately, our hope is that this book helps parents to feel more confident and empowered to help their child's sleep problem – so the whole family can get a better night's sleep.

Introduction

This book is split into three parts – in Part I we have provided you with information about children's sleep, including what sleep 'looks like'; how to tell if your child has a sleep problem; how sleep problems may develop, and how sleep and anxiety are related.

In Part II we take you through step-by-step techniques so you can support your child to overcome their sleep problem. This section is focused on sleep problems that are related to anxiety – such as when a child cannot fall asleep without a parent present, is very resistant to going to sleep, or perhaps needs to sleep in their parents' bed. We start by explaining two sleep techniques that are for use with children who have a lot of difficulty falling asleep, either when they first go to bed or when they wake during the night, without a parent or carer present. The first sleep technique we discuss is bedtime restriction (perhaps a slightly alarming name for what is a relatively straight-forward technique!). Next we describe a similar technique, referred to as sleep restriction. These treatments, which we have used with hundreds of families across our clinical and research work, are designed to take only a few weeks to implement (for some families, their child's sleep problem is fixed in as little as one week) and are our recommended first steps to improving your child's sleep. They are particularly designed to improve the quality of your child's sleep – helping them fall asleep faster and stay asleep during the night. In many cases we have found that these short treatments are enough to eliminate children's sleep problems.

However, we know that very anxious children may need some additional support. Therefore, Part II also provides step-by-step information on supporting your child to face their fears. First, for parents of older children (as a guide, 8+ years old), we explain how to help your child understand and challenge their fears and worries. Next we explain how to support children of any age to face their fears, one step at a time.

While the focus of these techniques is on children who are anxious about sleeping alone, we know that there are other sleep problems experienced by many children – including night terrors, sleep-walking and bed-wetting (a group of issues referred to as 'parasomnias'). Therefore, in Part III we focus on what to do to help your child with parasomnias. Again, we provide step-by-step guides to managing these issues.

Finally, even after your child's sleep has improved, it is important to remember no one sleeps perfectly all of the time (I'm sure we can all relate to that!). There may be 'blips' where you notice your child is falling back into poor sleep patterns. Therefore, in Part III we have also provided an overview of tips and tricks for helping your child maintain good sleep, including as they become a teenager.

Abbreviations

We will refer to some important abbreviations in this book. We'll remind you of their meaning throughout. We use the same acronyms that we use in our research and clinical work, as we know that some parents like to do further reading of research studies (e.g. search on Google Scholar), and we want parents to feel empowered to do so. To do this, though, it is important to know the correct terminology. We have provided the relevant definitions here, at the start of the book, so you can easily come back to them if necessary.

SOL = **S**leep **O**nset **L**atency: which is the amount of time it takes your child to fall asleep at the start of the night.

WASO = **W**ake **A**fter **S**leep **O**nset: which is the total amount of time that your child is awake for during the night (between falling asleep and before waking in the morning).

TST = **T**otal **S**leep **T**ime: which is the total amount of sleep they get overnight.

TIB = **T**ime **I**n **B**ed: which is the total amount of time between when you first put them to bed to sleep, and when they wake up and get out of bed the next day.

PART I

◇◇◇◇◇◇◇◇◇◇◇◇◇

Sleep: What It Looks Like, How Much, and Is It Enough?

What Does Sleep Look Like?

One of the first things we discuss with the families we see in our clinics is what sleep 'looks like'. We do this by drawing a graph on one of our whiteboards in our clinic rooms, just like the graph below (Figure 1). Understanding what sleep typically 'looks like' is an important step to understanding why your child has certain sleep problems and how you can help to target these problems.

Figure 1 shows a typical 9 hours of sleep for an average 'good' sleeper. The x-axis (horizontal line) represents the number of hours of sleep across the night, and the y-axis (vertical line) represents the depth of sleep. The lighter stages of sleep are higher on the graph, and the deeper stages of sleep are lower on the graph. Many people believe that when we fall asleep we go into a deep sleep, which lasts a few hours, and then gradually we surface in the morning. However, this is not true. You can see from Figure 1 that during sleep we go through many 'sleep cycles'. This is why, when we explain sleep to children, we say sleep is like a rollercoaster. Sleep cycles last about 90 minutes (or 1½ hours) or so, and we have several of them a night. Within these cycles you can see that it is perfectly normal to have periods of waking during the night. You might notice that your child's night-time wakings match these sleep cycles – that is, they wake at a time that matches an approximate 90-minute cycle (1½ hours after they fall asleep, 3 hours after they fall asleep, 4½ hours, 6 hours, etc.). This means they are likely waking from their lighter sleep stages. Of course, while short periods of waking are normal, night-time waking can be problematic (1) if they are unable to fall back to sleep, or (2) if they wake too many times. Or perhaps your child is able to fall back asleep, but only if you are present in their bedroom, or they are in your bed.

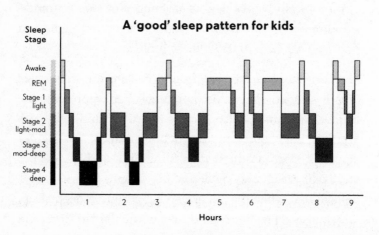

Figure 1 *Different stages of sleep across the night for school-aged children.*

What about the other stages of sleep? Near the 'waking' stages of Figure 1, you will notice a stage of sleep called 'REM sleep'. REM stands for 'rapid eye movement', which is exactly what happens during this stage of sleep. Our eyes are darting around under our eyelids. Not only that, but we are breathing more rapidly, our heart is beating faster and, importantly, there is a lot of brain activity. In fact, the brain activity that occurs during REM sleep might look similar to your brain activity right now. What is our mind doing during REM sleep? If you wake someone up from REM sleep, they are more likely to report having just dreamed. Yet, luckily there is another unique characteristic about REM sleep. Our muscles are paralysed – and for good reason. Because if they weren't, then we would act out our dreams. Now on the one hand that might sound exciting, but on the other hand there are people who have a sleep disorder known as 'REM Sleep Behaviour Disorder', and when they act out their dreams it can actually cause them physical harm. For example, one adult we saw several years ago reported a dream of being chased. This dream occurred on a regular basis. While he was still in his dream state, he physically got up out of bed, ran out of the bedroom, and literally ran through the back door, smashing through the glass. But even that did not wake him up. From this example you can clearly see that muscle paralysis can be very protective. REM sleep is paradoxical: it is an active stage of sleep, yet we still remain asleep.

Now imagine your child waking up from REM sleep, regardless of if they remember their dreams or not. Your child's heart may be racing, they are breathing a bit faster, and their mind is more active. Lying in the dark with all of those bodily sensations, imagine how difficult it may be for them to turn over and fall back to sleep. If your child wakes you during the night, remember that their mind and body might be quite active. This inevitably means that it might take their mind and body a while to relax enough to fall back to sleep. In this book we talk about some techniques that are designed to reduce the chance of your child experiencing these wakings altogether. And even if they do wake and are alert, we have additional techniques that can help them settle back to sleep – with practice.

> *'If your child wakes you during the night, remember that their mind and body might be quite active.'*

Finally, in Figure 1 you will see Stages 1–4, known as the 'non-REM' sleep stages. Of these stages, Stage 1 is the lightest sleep and Stage 4 the deepest. Stage 1 sleep is a very hard stage of sleep to detect because it is so light. Yet it is the beginning of us ignoring our surroundings. If woken from Stage 1 sleep, we may still recall sounds from our environment, even thoughts passing through our mind, but our memories start becoming poor. To explain this stage, we often provide the example of a parent dozing off during a movie. They might start breathing heavily or even lightly snoring. But being nudged to wake up, they insist that they were never asleep. They might even be able to remember some vague details about the movie. Stage 2 sleep is a more moderate depth of sleep, and a stage of sleep that we can have a lot of during the night (especially in the last half of the night). Stage 2 sleep may be best characterised by the sleep you wake from after a short nap. You may wake with a funny taste in your mouth, believing you did fall asleep, but that it wasn't a deep sleep. Finally, Stages 3 and 4 are deep stages of sleep. Stage 4 is a deeper sleep than Stage 3. Waking someone from these stages can be very difficult, especially a child. They might appear very drowsy or easily fall back to sleep.

You'll also notice in Figure 1 that most of the deep sleep occurs in the first half of the night. This is because deep sleep is related to a concept known as 'sleep pressure'. Sleep pressure ranks as one of the top two reasons for why and when we sleep (the other top reason is the timing of our internal body clock, known as the circadian rhythm). Sleep pressure is a biological process that begins to develop at 2 months of age, and occurs throughout our lifespan. The reason we are stressing this point is that if you understand how sleep pressure works, you can learn how to control sleep pressure in your child, such that they will fall asleep more quickly and be less likely to wake during the night. Sleep pressure is a key factor in the behavioural sleep techniques we discuss later in this book.

How Much Sleep Does My Child Need?

This is one of the questions we get asked most frequently by parents. Maybe their child doesn't seem to sleep as much as their sibling or as much as their peers, with the assumption being that less sleep might impact on their child's life. Many parents may hear via various media sources (e.g. TV, radio, etc.), that school-aged children should get something like 10 hours of sleep each night.

There are several research studies that have measured the sleep of thousands of school-aged children, usually using parent-reports (e.g. surveys asking parents to answer a question about their child's sleep, as opposed to a device like an activity-monitoring watch). These include the National Sleep Foundation polls from the United States (you can find these by typing 'national sleep foundation polls' into a search engine), surveys from Europe, Australia, and across the world. Many of these studies will provide the average amount of sleep that children of different ages get. And it is the average that people tend to focus on. In reality, the sleep needs of children differ between individual children – just as height, shoe size, and weight varies. For example, for an 8-year-old child, the mean amount of sleep obtained is roughly 10 hours, but about 80 per cent of all 8 year olds obtain 9 to 11 hours. Getting less sleep does not always equal a sleep problem. We encourage parents not to focus too much on the amount of sleep their child is getting, rather on the *quality* of that sleep – and, crucially, how their child functions during the day. Thus, your child may not have a serious sleep problem because the sleep that they are getting at night is enough for them to function fine during the day. All humans vary in the amount of sleep we get, and we all vary in how much sleep we need.

'We encourage parents not to focus too much on the amount of sleep their child is getting, rather on the quality *of that sleep – and, crucially, how their child functions during the day.'*

Figure 2 shows a 'bell curve' of children's sleep quantity. A bell curve shows the normal distribution of a particular measurement. On the y-axis is the number of children, and on the x-axis is the hours of sleep. Imagine that under this curve is a general population of 11 year olds. On average an 11-year-old child may need 10 hours' sleep. However, there will be some children of the same age who need 12 hours' sleep, and some who only need 8 hours' sleep. Sleep needs can differ dramatically between individuals of any age. We have even worked with adults who need as little as 2–3 hours of sleep!

When we explain this to children, we often use the example of height. About 60–70 per cent of all children of any particular age group will be in the 'average height' range. The curve is lower on the right-hand side because there are fewer really tall kids. And this is the same for really short kids. Children can often identify with this example as they can think of the tallest and shortest child in their class or grade level or school year group.

You might want to use this example to talk to your child about how much sleep they are getting, especially if they are worried that they are not sleeping enough or are sleeping too long. However, often we find that it is parents who find this information most useful, if they are feeling worried that their child may not be getting enough sleep.

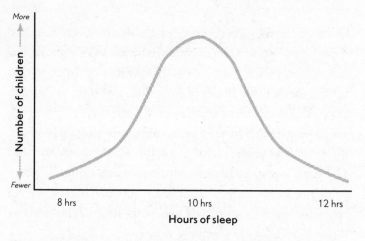

Figure 2 *A bell curve graph showing most children get 10 hours' sleep, whilst fewer children get 8 or 12 hours' sleep.*

So How Do You Know If Your Child Is Getting Enough Sleep?

The best way to determine if your child gets enough sleep is to look at how they function during the day. Are they functioning fine? Here we avoid using the phrase 'optimal functioning', because most people – children included – rarely function optimally each and every day of the week. As long as your child can function fine at school (and before and after school), then they are likely getting enough sleep to meet their needs.

If you answered that your child does not function fine during the day, then you have either observed them not functioning well in the morning before school, when they come home from school, and/or been informed by their teachers that they are not functioning well at school (maybe that they appear tired). Below is a list of some consequences children can experience from not sleeping well. Not all children will experience all of these – again, schoolchildren vary in their response to not getting enough sleep. Regardless of whether your child has one or more of these, what matters more is how much this is impacting on their life – and yours:

Some Consequences of Children Not Meeting Their Sleep Need

In the morning

- Hard to get out of bed

- Hard to wake up (falling back to sleep)

- Feeling tired and/or sleepy

- Feeling irritable and/or grumpy

- Lack of appetite for breakfast

- Not focused on getting ready for school

- Feeling unwell (headache, stomach-ache)

At school

- Difficulty concentrating

- Difficulty remembering information

- Feeling sleepy, tired, and/or grumpy

- Schoolwork and performance at school getting worse

- Not socialising as much as usual

- Aggression towards objects and others

- Constant yawning

After school

- Feeling flat and unmotivated

- Wanting to lie down or crawl into bed

- Actually falling asleep and napping

- Unwillingness to engage in activities

Importantly, even if your child is getting enough sleep, they can still have a sleep problem. Indeed, many of the children we see in our clinic are getting enough sleep and can function fine during the day. However, night-times are plagued by high levels of anxiety, or the child may be unable to sleep alone.

How to Tell If Your Child Has a Sleep Problem

If you're reading this book, then chances are that you already suspect your child has a sleep problem. Child sleep expert, Dr Richard Ferber, once mentioned that a sleep problem can be diagnosed by not only a health professional, but also by the child's parents. We agree with this view – parents are usually the best judges of whether their child has a sleep problem. Some of the signs of sleep problems include those in bullet points below. Of course, it is completely normal to sometimes have trouble sleeping (for children and adults). As we mentioned above, no one's sleep is perfect all of the time. However, if the problems listed below occur multiple nights per week, and last for months, this can indicate that your child has a sleep problem.

Problematic Night-Time Behaviours (When Persistent)

- Resisting or stalling to avoid going to bed

- Anxious at night and/or anxious about going to bed

- Needing a parent or sibling in their bedroom in order to sleep

- Wanting a parent awake and near their bedroom (e.g. in the next room) in order for them to fall asleep

- Sleeping in the parents'/parent's bed or bedroom (e.g. a mattress on the floor)

- Taking a long time to fall asleep (as a guide – longer than 20 minutes)

- Getting up and down from bed after you've put them to bed

- Waking a lot during the night (needing parents to help them fall back to sleep)

- Waking up during the night to go to sleep in the parents'/parent's bed or bedroom

- Anxious about sleeping away from home (e.g. sleeping over at a grandparent's or friend's house; going on a school camp)

There are also some unusual behaviours that can occur after the child has fallen asleep. During the night, some children may sleep-walk, some may wet the bed, and others can begin screaming, yet do not respond to a parent's comfort (night terrors). This collection of behaviours are known as 'parasomnias' (and we will also cover these in Part III).

What Are Common Sleep Problems for Children?

All children will likely go through periods where their sleep is not as good as usual. They may be anxious about something at school. There may be difficulties or extra stress in the home (like parental separation). They may even have seen something scary on television. However, in some cases these problems can persist for months and can begin to have a serious impact on family life, especially around night-time. We often see parents who must lie in bed with their child for hours until they fall asleep, or who have spent many years with their child asleep in their bed or in their bedroom. Child sleep problems can be particularly exhausting and time consuming for parents to manage. However, help is available in this book and our strategies can be used to make big improvements in your child's sleep. First, though, it is important to understand what the sleep problem is. Below we describe different types of sleep problems.

Insomnia

When a child has significant difficulty falling asleep and/ or staying asleep, and suffers daytime consequences because of their poor sleep, it is referred to as insomnia. For children, it can sometimes be referred to as 'behavioural insomnia' or 'insomnia of childhood'. For insomnia to be formally diagnosed, the problem needs to persist over several nights per week (at least three nights per week) and have been ongoing for a number of months (at least three months; American Academy of Sleep Medicine, 2014). In children, we typically see insomnia stemming from anxiety. The child might refuse to go to sleep unless a parent is lying with them or they are in their parents' bed, or they might wake up and not return to sleep unless a parent goes to them or they can sleep in their parents' bed. Parents often describe night-time as being particularly stressful – with their child getting very distressed and anxious at even the mention of going to sleep without the parent with them.

Below are two case studies of children who are experiencing insomnia during their middle childhood years.

THOMAS (10 YEARS OLD)

Thomas is a 10-year-old boy who takes a long time to fall asleep. Thomas's mum remembers that he has slept poorly since he was a toddler. When he was younger he would frequently get out of bed and end up sleeping in bed with his mum. He went through a period of time where he would fall asleep quite quickly if his mum lay down with him. If his mum suggested he go to sleep on his own, even if they checked the wardrobe and under the bed for monsters, or promised to check in on him, he would become very distressed. By around 8 years old Thomas would go to bed by himself, but would then be up and down many times until he either fell asleep or his mum went and sat with him. He found it hard to say what he was worried about but sometimes mentioned that he was worried that he would be taken by a robber. Night-times were often characterised by Thomas getting more and more upset as he wanted his mum to lie with him. While he generally stays asleep once he's fallen asleep, it now takes Thomas up to an hour to fall asleep each night – sometimes longer. His mum is finding that the night-time routine is taking up almost the whole evening, and Thomas still becomes very teary and clingy if she tries to suggest any changes. Of course, she also finds it very distressing to see Thomas so upset around bedtime. He is also becoming increasingly tired during the day and will often nap in the car on the way to school. Thomas often tells his mum that at night he has very bad dreams.

SOPHIE (6 YEARS OLD)

Sophie is a 6-year-old girl. She has a lot of trouble fall-ing asleep on her own and will flat out refuse to go to sleep unless her parent is with her. Sophie also wakes up frequently during the night, especially when she's put to sleep in her own bed. She shares a bedroom with her young brother and was starting to wake him up too. Therefore, to manage this and to help make sure that Sophie gets enough sleep, she now sleeps most nights in her parents' bed. Her mum or dad usually lie with her for at least an hour until she falls asleep. Recently her parents have trialled a mattress on their floor where Sophie now sleeps. A few times they have tried to move Sophie back to her own bed before they go to sleep, but she will usually wake during the night and come back to their room, and most mornings they will find her asleep on the mattress or at the end of their bed.

We will revisit these case studies in Part II when we pro-vide step-by-step techniques to help them sleep better.

Parasomnias

Parasomnias are a group of sleep problems that are cate-gorised as unusual or unwanted experiences, which occur when people are sleeping. In children, perhaps the most common parasomnias are bed-wetting, night terrors and sleep-walking. These unusual behaviours occur due to a clash between deep sleep and a burst of activity in the body. As such, the child will be in a state of awareness that lies between sleeping and waking. Some of these behaviours can be quite distressing to watch, but fortunately the child is not aware of them and does not recall them the following morning. It is important to keep the child safe during the events, and later in this book we will teach you a couple of techniques that may reduce the frequency and severity of parasomnias.

Below we present a case of a young boy with parasomnias. While this boy's particular parasomnia is night terrors, his treatment could apply to bed-wetting or sleep-walking.

HARRY (8 YEARS OLD)

Harry is an 8-year-old boy and experiences night terrors most nights. He usually falls asleep okay but often wakes up during the night, screaming as if he is being attacked. His parents recall that night terrors first began when he was a toddler. At first they thought he would grow out of it, but the terrors have persisted for a number of years and his parents have noticed that he is beginning to get very worried about falling asleep at night. Harry falls asleep around 7.30 p.m. each night and his night terrors usually happen about 9.30 p.m. – about 2 hours after he falls asleep.

We will discuss Harry and his sleep later in the book (Part III) where we will provide a couple of simple techniques that can be used to deal with this distressing sleep problem.

4

Understanding Sleep and Anxiety

Not all sleep problems stem from anxiety. For example, parasomnias like night terrors or bed-wetting are often not anxiety responses. However, the majority of cases we see are about children being very anxious or frightened to sleep alone. This is also a very common concern expressed to family doctors or general practitioners. Therefore, in this chapter, we want to provide you with more detail about the relationship between anxiety and sleep.

When the sleep clinic doors opened over a decade ago to see children with sleep problems, we did not know what to expect. After a year, we saw the same issues arise again and again. These kids were so anxious at night that they needed their parents nearby in order to sleep.

Sometimes this meant that children were sleeping in the same bedroom as their parents, even the same bed. Sometimes Mum or Dad could not go to bed, or begin to unwind, until their child fell asleep in the child's room with them nearby. Other times, parents would be woken during the night by the child walking (sometimes running) into the parents' bedroom. Sometimes parents would wake, startled, with a shadow looming over them (and seconds later realise it was their own child – not an intruder). And then other times, the parent would wake to find that the child had somehow managed to get into their bed without them knowing.

This was the sleep of the anxious child.

To our surprise, most of these children did not experience significant anxiety during the day. For example, they were able to separate from their parents at other times (such as going to school). However, these same children found it very difficult to separate from their parents at night. So there was something specific about their anxiety as bed-time approached.

Get in the Ring: Sleep and Anxiety As Opponents

Anxiety and The Three Fs

In the red corner, weighing over 200 kilograms, and with a record of disturbing over 1,200 nights, raise your hands for . . . Anxiety!

Anxiety is a normal and common emotion. We can all experience anxiety at times. However, anxiety can become a problem when it starts to impact on your child's life, for example in their ability to feel safe falling asleep in their own bed.

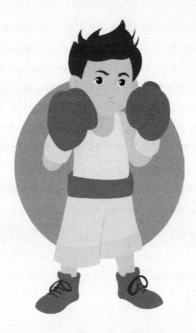

Anxiety is a formidable opponent of sleep. When your child sees or hears something scary, or even thinks of something scary, their body produces chemicals like adrenaline and cortisol (the 'stress hormone') to prepare them to react. We often refer to these reactions as the three Fs – *Fight*, *Flight* or *Freeze*. When a child experiences at least one of the three Fs, their heart begins to beat fast and pumps blood to where they need it most (e.g. their muscles) so they can run (Flight) or defend themselves (Fight). This also requires their lungs to pump more oxygen so it can be distributed through their blood to supply their muscles. Their bodies physiologically react as though they are in a threatening or dangerous situation, even if they are not.

As an example of the three Fs, imagine you are sitting in a work meeting on a quiet afternoon. A manager is speaking about recent developments in the workplace. In the middle of this meeting your colleague's phone rings. He answers the phone and quietly whispers, '*I'm in a meeting, I'll call you back*', and hangs up. This might be an interaction you have seen many times. You don't think anything of it. Then you notice the manager quietly strolling over to your colleague. They take your colleague's phone and proceed to smash it against the desk – again and again and again.

How would your body react to this alarming and unexpected event? Would your heart start beating faster? Would you freeze, not knowing what to do? Would you quickly leave the room?

Well this is an example where the three Fs could work.

First is Freeze. Many people would feel frightened at this sudden outburst and might freeze or feel unable to move or say anything. Second is Flight. Some people may be so alarmed at the person's actions that they would flee the room. Third and finally is Fight. Some people may be so angry at the manager's behaviour (perhaps, in this case, the person who owned the phone), that they would begin to argue with the manager.[1]

---

1   We should note here that this scenario is adapted from a novel 'classroom experiment' performed each year on unsuspecting university students by sleep expert Professor Leon Lack at Flinders University, who taught biological psychology. Of course, the phone was fake and the student who answered the phone was a stooge.

Any of these behaviours may be a reaction to an alarming event. And this alarming event is an obvious one (i.e. it was unexpected and aggressive). However, for your child, the alarming event can be much more subtle. A common event, or trigger, we hear from children with a sleep problem is a noise they heard outside when it was night-time. Whilst, as adults, we can quickly work out what was likely to have made a noise outside, some children cannot, and may begin to think of the worst thing (e.g. it's an intruder). This 'event' may trigger the three Fs in your child. A Freeze reaction might be your child lying very still, not being able to sleep. A Flight reaction might be your child running to you or your bedroom to seek reassurance. A Fight reaction might mean them screaming or yelling at you as they resist going back into their bedroom where they feel afraid.

For some children the three Fs may even be triggered by the very 'event' of going to bed. If they are worried about monsters or a scary character they have seen, scared about a frightening story they heard, scared about themselves or their family dying or worried about being away from their parent, going to their bed can actually trigger the three Fs. Bed is where they worry about being alone and where they have space to think about scary things, or hear all of those noises outside. Typically, for these children, the very thought of bed causes either a Fight (e.g. arguing) or Flight (e.g. refusing to stay in bed) response.

To understand the impact of anxiety and the three Fs on sleep, the most important reactions to be aware of are alertness or hyper-vigilance. Hyper-vigilance means that a person appears 'on guard', constantly assessing their surroundings for any threat or danger, and constantly picking up on any slight suggestion that their fear is going to come true – this is obviously not a helpful state for the body to be in while it is trying to get to sleep.

To sum it up:

- Children with a sleep problem are likely to be awake in bed

- An event (e.g. hearing a noise outside) or even the thought of going to bed can trigger anxiety, leading to the three Fs (Freeze, Fight, Flight)

- Any one of the three Fs increases children's physiological arousal (e.g. increased heart rate)

- Importantly, the three Fs result in your child being very alert at night

- Being anxious and hyper-vigilant at night is the opponent of sleep . . .

And Here Comes Sleep!

In the blue corner, weighing more and more kilograms the more time passes by, and with a world record of over 3,500 nights of slumber, raise your hands for . . . Sleep!

After the above description of what anxiety can do to our bodies and minds, one would think that sleep has no chance of winning. In fact, time and time again you have probably experienced yourself that your child's anxiety wins the fight over sleep. But we want to reassure you that this does not have to be the case. Sleep is an evolutionary need. No matter how long people try to stay awake, sleep will eventually occur. Thus, sleep is very powerful indeed.

Anxiety can make it very difficult to sleep – the physiological responses produced in our body when we are anxious or scared (the three Fs) act as a direct opponent of sleep. Despite all this, the need to sleep will eventually win. For example, ask yourself how many nights your child has had an all-nighter – where they have not fallen asleep at all. For many it will never have happened, or maybe just a few times. Now think about how many nights your child had *some* sleep in a given year. We are sure that the nights that they got at least some sleep (no matter how anxious they were) far outweigh any nights where they had no sleep (or even only a few hours' sleep). So, no matter how much or how long someone tries to fight off sleep, eventually sleep wins and people will sleep. Adults have tried to go without sleep for days in a row and, before they know it, they lose. Even little bits of sleep, known as 'micro-sleeps', occur when trying not to sleep (e.g. when someone is very sleepy and is sitting quietly watching the TV or a movie). These micro-sleeps sneak in, even when people have their eyes open. For children, it is even harder to try and fight off sleep.

Sleep is a Ninja

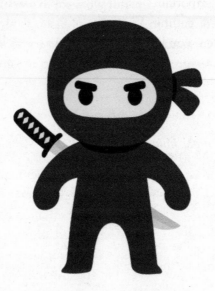

In our opinion, sleep is not a metaphorical boxer trying to combat anxiety head-on. Sleep is a ninja. And a good ninja at that. Sleep creeps up on you without you knowing it. It's silent and stealthy. And no matter how hard you try (and we've met some kids that have tried *very* hard!), sleep always wins. So when going into battle with anxiety, the sleep ninja is the sort of ally you want on your side.

At the start of this section we mentioned that sleep and anxiety are related in important ways. Sleep and anxiety are opponents. As much as 'Anxiety the Boxer' looks fierce, at the end of the day, the 'Sleep Ninja' wins. Metaphors aside, here's the science.

The longer humans stay awake, the sleepier they get. This is an important 'take-home message'. You may have experienced getting gradually sleepier and sleepier on nights where you have had to stay up late. This is known as sleep pressure; it is a concept we briefly introduced in Part I, chapter 1, and one which we describe in more detail in Part II.

> 'The longer humans stay awake, the sleepier they get.'

One theory, proposed by researchers Ronald Dahl and Allison Harvey, which supports what we see in our clinical work, is the possibility that sleepiness can dampen anxiety. That is, the longer children stay awake, the more sleep pressure builds. The more sleepy children get in the evening, the less they care about the things that go bump in the night. Our own and others' research has provided some support for this idea, finding that simply allowing children to stay up later and get sleepier in the evening has led to them reporting less anxiety.

However, there could be another important way in which children become less anxious due to the sleep techniques we use (and will teach you). That is, lying in bed when your child is not ready to sleep can create the perfect environment for worry.

Most parents hear of the importance of children (indeed everyone) getting enough sleep. So, when trying to work out what time your child should go to bed, a bit of mathematics follows. That is, you know when your child needs to get up for school so, working backwards, you estimate when they should go to bed in order to get enough sleep. Another way of determining their bedtime is by hearing about when other children their age go to bed, and then setting this bedtime for your child. However, not all children are built the same. Earlier, in Part I, chapter 1, we explained that lots of children get the same amount of sleep, yet a few children seem to need less. If a child does not need as much sleep as their friends, they will also naturally fall asleep later than their friends. If they are still put to bed at the same time as their friends, they may be lying awake until their body is ready for sleep. This is far from ideal. It is night-time; it's dark and quiet. This provides a great opportunity for children to be hyper-vigilant of their surroundings and, in turn, hyper-vigilant to the thoughts and worries that rush through their minds. Combine a child's imagination, the things they have seen or heard about, with lying down in bed in the dark, and a noise outside, and it is no wonder that children become anxious in bed.

Thus, the second important way that anxiety and sleep are related is that children can become anxious when they are awake in bed. And we know, at least from studies in adults, that a racing mind is more likely to occur in the evening. Thus, being awake in bed, unable to sleep, provides a perfect opportunity for children to worry. This was another theory proposed by Professors Dahl and Harvey. And it is also a theory we tested in our research. To test this, we limited the opportunity for anxious children to be awake in bed during the night, using simple behavioural techniques that we describe in Part II. As a result, we observed that, after only a couple of weeks, they became less anxious and were falling asleep far quicker.

> *'Being awake in bed, unable to sleep, provides a perfect opportunity for children to worry.'*

Summing It Up

There are two important ways sleep and anxiety are related in children:

1. Sleep and anxiety are opponents (the ninja v. the boxer).

2. Lying awake during the night allows children to worry. If we reduce this opportunity to worry, then anxiety begins to reduce and your child learns they can fall asleep safely in their bed.

With point 1 above, we know that when anxiety is high, sleepiness is low. Yet if we build up sleepiness, it will eventually overcome anxiety. With this in mind, it can be possible to dampen anxiety by increasing sleepiness. In Part II, we provide simple step-by-step behavioural strategies that you can use to help build up sleepiness in your anxious child.

So my child will be less anxious at night but get sleepy during the day, we hear you say?

No. Importantly, our studies have found that, when done right, these techniques can increase sleepiness in the evening, yet have little to no impact on children's functioning during the day.

> *'We know that when anxiety is high, sleepiness is low. Yet if we build up sleepiness, it will eventually overcome anxiety.'*

As outlined in point 2 and above, if we reduce the opportunity to worry, then anxiety begins to reduce, and children learn that they do not have to be worried about sleeping in their own bed at night-time. The way we reduce the opportunity to worry is to limit the amount of time children spend awake in bed during the night.

In Part II of this book, we provide step-by-step guidance on how to implement simple behavioural techniques to help limit your child's worrying in bed.

5

How Do Sleep Problems Develop and Why Do They Stick Around?

The Three Ps

Unlike the three Fs, the three Ps are a little harder to remember. They stand for:

1. **P**redisposing factors (*things the child is born with*)

2. **P**recipitating factors (*stressful events*)

3. **P**erpetuating factors (*thoughts and behaviours that continue the problem*)

The three Ps can help us understand how sleep problems develop and stick around in children.

Factors That Predispose Children to Developing a Sleep Problem

It is likely that sleep problems in children develop for a combination of reasons. 'Predisposing factors' are things that the child is born with (e.g. genetics, temperament) that make them more or less likely to develop a sleep problem. Predisposing factors are not necessarily the only cause of a sleep problem – it's more like they give a sleep problem a head start. First, some children have genes that increase the chances of developing a sleep problem. It could be as simple as genetically not needing much sleep, or genetically being a 'night owl' (i.e., they naturally fall asleep later than the average child their age). Closely related to this is that some children are born with a temperament that is strong-willed so, despite parents' best efforts to manage boundaries around their child's behaviours at night, such children often 'win' enough of these battles. There are a number of other factors that can increase the chances of a child developing a sleep problem, including being an 'over-thinker' or a 'worrier', being more susceptible to becoming anxious. There might be a family history of 'worriers', anxiety, or sleep difficulties.

> *'Predisposing factors are things that the child is born with (e.g. genetics, temperament) that make them more or less likely to develop a sleep problem.'*

One predisposing factor mentioned in the adult scientific literature is vulnerability to stress. Like height, weight, and sleep need, we can all differ in how vulnerable we are to stress. The phrase 'water off a duck's back' can sometimes refer to people who are largely unaffected by stress. At the other end, there can be people who some would consider to 'overreact' to stress, or find stress more difficult to deal with.

On their own, predisposing factors are not the only cause of a child's sleep problem. They generally need to be combined with other factors, stacked on top of them, to cause the child to develop a sleep problem.

Stress and Stressful Events that Trigger Sleep Difficulties

'Precipitating factors' are stressful events that can suddenly trigger bad sleep. Some examples of precipitating factors include:

- death of a loved one (including a pet)

- parental separation

- being bullied at school

- having an accident and/or hospitalisation

- being ill

- watching a scary movie

When you add a precipitating event to predisposing factors, the combination of these two Ps can cause a child to develop a sleep problem. This is actually pretty normal, as most people who experience a stressful event will sleep badly for a while but the problem will soon resolve. It is expected over time that the stressful event can resolve itself, so that it is not so bad. But, there is now a third and final 'P' factor. And the addition of this final factor can determine whether a child *continues* to have a sleep problem or not.

> 'Precipitating factors are stressful events that can suddenly trigger bad sleep.'

Factors that Maintain a Child's Sleep Problem

'Perpetuating factors' are typically thoughts, emotions and behaviours that maintain a child's sleep problem. These mainly come from within the child, but can also be influenced by how the parent responds to the child's anxiety or behaviour. Perpetuating factors can emerge around the time of the stressful event, and grow as time goes on.

In our clinical work we also often see that a cycle can develop, where actions taken to help children sleep better may have inadvertently maintained the sleep problem. Of course, parents do not like to see their child distressed, and night-times can be a particularly difficult time to manage your child's anxiety – they are tired, you are tired; everyone's ability to tolerate the child's distress may be reduced. Nevertheless, we know from sleep and anxiety research that parents' responses can unknowingly maintain the problem. One way that parents can unknowingly maintain their child's night-time anxiety is by allowing the child to avoid what they are afraid of (i.e. sleeping alone in their own bed). To ensure their child sleeps, the parent may have developed a routine whereby they will either go to bed and lie with the child until they fall asleep, or where the child sleeps in the parent's/parents' bed or bedroom. This certainly provides a short-term solution as it removes the child from the situation where they experienced anxiety and allows them to go to sleep. However, it is rarely a long-term solution and can actually act to heighten the belief that their bed is not a safe place for them (see the 'sleep anxiety cycle' below; Figure 3).

> *'Perpetuating factors are typically thoughts, emotions and behaviours that maintain a child's sleep problem.'*

At many points of the sleep anxiety cycle, both the child and parent are rewarded. For both the child and parent, the first reward is that the child's anxiety is reduced, while the second reward is that the child is able to fall asleep. A further reward for the parent may be that they are then able to relax as they have not had to manage the child's bedtime resistance and their child has fallen asleep. And what we know from rewarding behaviour is that the behaviour is likely to recur (in this case, the following night). However, it also means that the child does not have the opportunity to begin learning that they can be safe sleeping in their bed. Breaking this cycle is something we cover in this book, via a technique called 'Exposure' (see Part II, chapter 5).

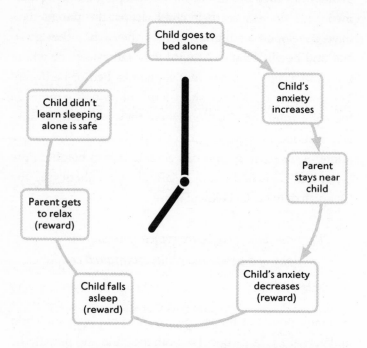

Figure 3 *The 'sleep anxiety cycle', which continues every night unless broken by some of the techniques taught in Part II.*

Besides avoiding the feared situation, many parents we see go to great lengths to try to reassure their child that there is nothing to be anxious about. Bedtime may become a time of lots of conversation and the child seeking reassurance from their parents. At bedtime, reassurance-seeking might involve your child frequently calling out from their bed to make sure you are there, asking you to check outside repeatedly to see that there are no intruders, asking that you sit with them in bed. It might involve your child wanting to engage in a conversation about lots of different worries. While it is important that your child can have space to talk about their feelings and worries, bedtime is not necessarily the best time for this.

Like avoidance, seeking reassurance is an understandable reaction to anxiety. Children often look to their parents to help them make sense of what is going on or to seek comfort, and parents naturally want to comfort their child. However, from the anxiety literature, we know that seeking reassurance over and over again about the same situation (i.e. going to bed) can be an unhelpful way of coping. Giving reassurance – always responding, sitting with them, going outside to 'check' for intruders – might be a way of immediately relieving your child's anxiety, but in the longer term we know that it can maintain the very anxiety that the parent is trying to calm. Over-reassurance sends a message that there is an actual danger at night-time that they need to be protected from. It can actually confirm to the child that they are indeed not safe.

Spotting the Three Ps

Eleven-year old Trinity has always been a bit of a thinker, and focuses a lot on what's going on in the news. She goes on a holiday with her family for a couple of weeks, where the whole family sleep in the same room. She has a great time and her sleep has also been great. When the family returns home, and Trinity goes to her own bed, suddenly she is wide awake at night, and frequently complains to her parents each night that she isn't tired. After a few nights of this, she becomes distressed, and after a very late night, Trinity's mum makes her sleep with her in the parents' bed so that she gets some rest. Trinity falls asleep very quickly. The next night Trinity asks to sleep in her mum's bed, and despite Mum refusing, the night again turns into a late one, full of tears, and eventually Mum allows Trinity to come into her bed so she can get enough sleep (as Trinity has school the next day). This pattern repeats itself for the remainder of the school week. At the weekend, Trinity has a friend to sleep over. They both have a late night, but both of them fall asleep fine in Trinity's bedroom. The next night, Trinity asks her mum if she can sleep in her bed again.

Did you spot the three Ps?

The predisposing factors were in the first sentence – Trinity is the type of child who is alert to her surroundings and doesn't switch off easily.

How about the precipitating factor – that is, the event that triggered the sleep problem? In this example, this may be a little harder to spot. In this example, it was the change from sleeping with her family on holiday to going back home and sleeping independently in her own room.

Finally, did you spot the perpetuating factors? Trinity was in a 'new' environment (sleeping independently in her own room) and if an 'event' occurred (i.e. turning the lights off), this could then lead her to think about threats that occur in the dark (e.g. a robber), which would lead to emotions (anxiety, distress), and then behaviours (coming out of her bedroom saying she could not sleep/wanting to sleep in her parents' bed).

The other perpetuating factors were her parents allowing Trinity to sleep in their bed. As we have already alluded to, when parents are 'in the moment', when their child is distressed late at night and they have school the next morning, having their child sleep in their bed is a quick solution to the problem. Parents usually intend this to be temporary but, unfortunately, in some cases, it can teach children that in order to sleep they need the presence of their parents. Sometimes children occasionally sleep in their parents' bed but it is only temporary; for others, where there might be other precipitating or perpetuating factors involved, this can be the beginning of the development and maintenance of a longer-term sleep problem.

There are many different things that can lead to, or maintain, a child's sleep problem. They can be easy to spot if your child is able to tell you about them – for example, each year there seems to be a new scary character that children see or hear about on YouTube, in videogames, movies, or hear about from their friends. *Bloody Mary*, *Slender Man*, *Five Nights at Freddy's*, and clowns roaming the streets, are a few examples that send many families to see us. If a child hears a noise outside at night, the child may quickly surmise that it is one of these scary characters making that noise. So the child won't stay in their bedroom alone, and will seek security from their parents.

Sometimes the precipitating event has not occurred, but a thought about a future event frightens children. We see many school-aged children who are about to go on a school camp or residential trips. The thought of going camping away from their parent/parents can trigger a stressful response in the child; in turn, they have great trouble sleeping. Many children are scared of not having their parent/parents accessible 'if something goes wrong' when they are at camp. No matter what the precipitating factor may be – in most cases you can see that the child is seeking comfort and safety from their parent.

> *'The thought of going camping away from their parent/parents can trigger a stressful response in the child; in turn, they have great trouble sleeping.'*

While it is possible that children with sleep problems can get better by themselves, this is generally considered rare once a sleep disorder has been established (i.e. where the problem occurs for three or more nights per week and for a number of months). For example, we found that out of twenty children on a two-month waiting list at our sleep clinic, only one child (5 per cent) got better without any intervention.

We understand that being a parent of a child with a sleep problem is a tough thing to deal with every single day (and night). Therefore, the sooner you can understand the techniques to help your child's sleep problem, the better they will feel, and the better you will feel.

Are You Ready?

It is really important to be committed to following a sleep programme through to the end. Persistence and consistency are keys to an effective sleep intervention. Sometimes it can be helpful to consider whether *now* is the right time for you to do this.

One technique that can help is a list called a 'Decisional Balance Sheet', which is a fancy name for a 'List of Pros and Cons'. Here you can list what are the good things about your child's sleep problem (on the left-hand side of the sheet), and the things you don't like about your child's sleep problem (on the right-hand side of the sheet). We've entered examples on each side to help you get started.

Decisional Balance Sheet

Good Things *about my child's sleep problem*		**Not-so-good Things** *about my child's sleep problem*	
It's sometimes nice to have my child sleep in my bed – especially at weekends.	2	*My sleep is always broken – I just want to be able to sleep through again!*	5
Good Total		Not-So-Good Total	

Adapted from Miller & Rollnick (2012).

If you have managed to write some good things, and not-so-good things, we now ask you to write a number next to each one, where a 1 means *Not really important* and 5 means *Very important*. After you have done that, then add up the numbers on the good side, and enter the total in the 'good total' box. Then add the numbers up on the not-so-good side. Look below at where your motivation may be right now when it comes to making a change to your child's sleep problem:

The numbers only differ by 1 or are the same = You may not be ready to make a change. It may take longer for you to build motivation, or there may be a tipping point at which you have 'had enough' and it's time to make a change. It might be best for you to redo the Decisional Balance Sheet next week to see if your motivation has changed.

The 'good' score is bigger than the 'not-so-good' score = You are finding that the benefits of your child having a sleep difficulty outweigh the negatives of their sleep difficulty. This can happen for some families. As we point out in our example above, some parents enjoy having a child sleep in their bed when the other parent is away (e.g. for work), or parents are separated, or one parent snores (and thus sleeps in another room). This may stay this way, or circumstances might change (i.e. the child is 'ready' to move back to their own bedroom; you feel as though it's time for your child to sleep more independently). You may wish to redo the Decisional Balance Sheet again in a month's time to see if it is the right time to begin the intervention.

The 'not-so-good' score is bigger than the 'good' score =
This suggests you are ready to do one of the behavioural
or cognitive techniques you can learn from this book. As a
double-check, what number would you choose below?

*I **will** start my child's new sleep technique(s) within
the next three days*

Probably will   1   2   3   4   5   6   7   8   9   10   *Definitely will*

If you chose at least a 7, then there is an excellent chance
you are ready to prioritise helping your child to overcome
their sleep problem. If not, that is okay, but it is best to
wait until you are motivated enough to persist with the
techniques.

Sometimes, people need a goal to help motivate them and
be ready to make a change to their lives. So there may be
goals that come up in future, whether they are a family
holiday, a time when you would like your child to be able
to go on a school camp, on a sleepover to a friend's house,
or you may want to go on a late-night outing.

Please don't leave a sleep programme to the last minute!

Plan ahead – weeks ahead – and then you will give yourself and your child a better chance to enjoy successful and
restful sleep.

PART II

◇◇◇◇◇◇◇◇◇◇◇◇◇

1. The Roadmap to Helping Your Child with Sleep Problems

2. Preparing for a Sleep Intervention: Sleep Hygiene and Bedtime Routines, Myths and Misconceptions, Measuring Sleep, Setting Goals

3. Helping Your Child to Fall Asleep and Stay Asleep: Bedtime and Sleep Restriction

4. Helping Your Child to Understand and Challenge Their Night-Time Fears and Worries

5. Exposure: Helping Your Child to Face Their Fears Step By Step

6. Relaxation Techniques

1

The Roadmap to Helping Your Child with Sleep Problems

The most common sleep problems we see in our clinical work are children who experience anxiety around bedtime. They might want a parent to sit with them to fall asleep, only sleep in their parent's/parents' bed, or demonstrate a lot of refusal or resistance around bedtime. In Part II we provide step-by-step guides to implementing evidence-based sleep interventions for your child, which target these presentations. We provide two options – Bedtime Restriction and Sleep Restriction – which are both based on our clinical work and research done by ourselves and other groups, and are generally aimed at children aged 5–12 years old. While every child is unique, and sleep problems can vary, we have found that these techniques can be very effective for most children's sleep problems, where the problem is related to worry or anxiety. While either intervention is useful for these problems, at the end of this section you will find a roadmap designed to help you identify which intervention might best suit your child. Before beginning either Bedtime Restriction or Sleep Restriction, we would also recommend you read the opening of each intervention and decide which one will work best for you and your child (see Part II, chapter 3). If your main concern about your child's sleep is parasomnias (e.g. bed-wetting, night terrors, sleep-walking), please refer to Part III (as highlighted in the roadmap at the end of this section).

Add-On Components

For many children, two to three weeks using either Bedtime Restriction or Sleep Restriction will be enough to get their sleep back on track. We have seen many families who, after years of struggling with their child's sleep, are able to resolve the issue in only two weeks. However, in some cases children might continue to experience some night-time anxiety or continue to struggle to sleep without a parent present. This isn't anything to worry about, as there are further evidence-based techniques (which again only take a few weeks) that you can use to support your child to face their fears and worries. In cases where Bedtime Restriction or Sleep Restriction don't completely resolve the problem, older children (as a guide, 8+ years old) may also benefit from understanding more about how their thoughts and feelings impact on their behaviour, and in turn this will help them deal with their night-time anxiety. Cognitive techniques are a core component of many evidence-based psychological interventions for anxiety, and you will find these explained in detail in many excellent parent guides (e.g. *Helping Your Child with Fears and Worries* by Cathy Creswell and Lucy Willetts). Often cognitive techniques are not necessary for sleep interventions, where children experience significant gains from the behavioural sleep interventions (i.e. Bedtime Restriction or Sleep Restriction). However, we know that having a child who you may describe as an 'over-thinker', and having a child with a sleep problem, often go hand-in-hand. Therefore, we have included this section about helping your child to identify and overcome their worry thoughts (Part II, chapter 4) for parents who think their child may benefit from having this higher level of understanding of the processes that can maintain their fear or anxiety around bedtime.

For all children (regardless of age) who continue to experience anxiety after the first-step sleep intervention (Bedtime or Sleep Restriction), you should move on to the Exposure section, which provides a step-by-step guide for supporting your child to face their fears and overcome them (described later in Part II, chapter 5). Most commonly in our clinical practice, for children who experience night-time anxiety, we would begin with either Bedtime Restriction or Sleep Restriction, followed by Exposure.

> *'Most commonly in our clinical practice, for children who experience night-time anxiety, we would begin with either Bedtime Restriction or Sleep Restriction, followed by Exposure.'*

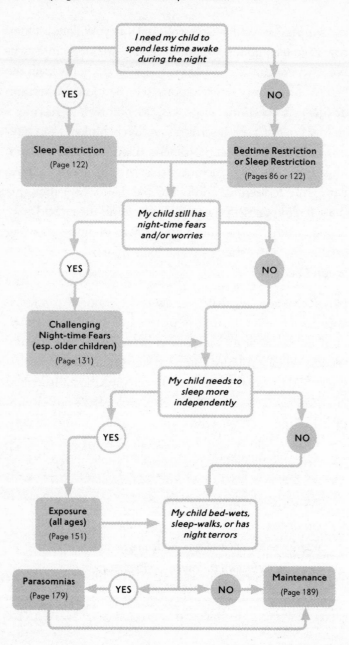

2

Preparing for a Sleep Intervention: Sleep Hygiene and Bedtime Routines, Myths and Misconceptions, Measuring Sleep, Setting Goals

Whichever sleep intervention you choose, the best scientific and clinical evidence we have is that to improve your child's sleep requires some change in their routine. Whichever sleep technique you try from this book, the first step will likely involve their bedtime being temporarily moved later (we will present examples of this in due course). This means for a (short) period of time, you may also be going to sleep later than usual and may feel more tired than usual. The phrase 'short-term pain for long-term gain' rings true across most evidence-based sleep interventions. The key to success with these programmes is remaining consistent and persevering. This can be difficult if you are also sleep deprived – if your child is having trouble sleeping, chances are that this has also affected your sleep. Therefore, to maximise the chance of success, it is important that you are prepared. Helping your child face their fears and worries inevitably means they are facing situations where they may at first feel upset. Therefore, if you can, it is ideal to have another adult (e.g. your partner, your own parent, a supportive friend) who can support you with this process. This is not to say that you cannot do these strategies on your own. We have worked with many single parents and caregivers who are able to successfully implement the strategies used in this book. However, some support from a relative or friend can go a long way to help you manage the sleep intervention. It's particularly important to inform others if your child stays at another house during their programme (e.g. with another parent or grandparent), so they can also stick to the programme as much as possible. You might even choose to tell their teacher if you decide to do a treatment programme that begins with some restriction of your child's sleep (more about this later). Overall, most sleep programmes take at least three weeks, so try to choose a period of time where you and your child will be able to stick to the changes in the sleep routine to ensure the best chance of success.

> *'Try to choose a period of time where you and your child will be able to stick to the changes in the sleep routine to ensure the best chance of success.'*

Sleep Hygiene: Giving Your Child the Best Chance to Fall Asleep

Before starting, it is important to make sure that your child's environment gives them the best chance to feel sleepy and fall asleep. This is commonly referred to as 'sleep hygiene'. These are factors that we know can help your child's brain and body get ready to sleep. A pre-sleep bedtime routine is an important step for getting ready to sleep. This includes having a consistent bedtime *and* wake-up time, as well as making sure your child's body has a chance to relax and unwind. Below are some key dos and don'ts for your child's pre-bed routine:

DO:

Let them:

- Have 'quiet time' for at least an hour before bedtime

- Keep lights as dim as possible

- Avoid *interactive* technology (e.g. gaming, social media)

- Avoid watching television programmes that may be overly stimulating – those that might make them feel scared or very excited, for example

- Avoid homework (or other activities) that may make them feel stressed

DON'T:

Let them:

- Nap after school

- Consume caffeinated beverages or food in the afternoon and evening

- Fall asleep anywhere except their bed

- Have a long hot bath or shower immediately before bed (especially if your child has some sensory sensitivity, like often complaining of feeling too hot). A long hot shower or bath can raise their internal body temperature, the opposite of what is needed for sleep

- Let your child use their bed for activities other than sleeping (e.g. homework, watching TV)

Making sure your child has a good bedtime routine is one relatively simple step you can take to ensure you are giving them the best chance of falling asleep. While you may not be able to stick to a bedtime routine all the time, having consistency around bedtime is a useful way of giving your child the best chance of success at sleeping. A bedtime routine should include all parts of getting ready for bed – such as brushing teeth, getting in pyjamas, and quiet activities like reading a book; whatever it is that needs to happen between dinner and bedtime to get your child prepared.

Of course, routines have to work for all family members, but do try to have at least an hour of 'wind-down' time before your child goes to bed. It may also be useful to consider the order in which things are done. For example, reading a book with your child is a lovely activity that can promote a range of benefits for their learning. A book in bed is a common part of bedtime routines. However, in our clinical work we have sometimes found that the bedtime book can actually create a source of anxiety, as the child anticipates when their parent is going to leave the room. Or they may use it as a chance to try to keep the parent with them – *'Just one more book, pleeeease.'* If you think this may be an issue for your child, we might recommend the night-time book be moved to the sofa, before your child gets into bed. This allows the routine of actually getting into bed to be kept as minimal as possible: into bed, tucked in, a kiss goodnight and that is all. Simple, right? Of course, it might not run that smoothly (at least at first). Nevertheless, these can be simple ways of making changes to reduce anxiety in the long run.

Chloe's bedtime routine

Chloe's bedtime is 8 p.m. The family aim to have dinner around 6 p.m. After dinner she has a quick shower. By around 7 p.m., Chloe begins her wind-down time. She brushes her teeth and gets in her pyjamas, ready to relax. She has her last glass of water for the day at least an hour before her bedtime. In her quiet time, Chloe does some drawing at the kitchen table or builds Lego with her sister. Sometimes she's allowed to watch TV. During her wind-down time, Chloe and her parent also always read a book together. Just before 8 p.m., Chloe is encouraged to go to the toilet. Her parents make sure Chloe's bedroom light is turned off but her night-light is on. At 8 p.m., Chloe is put to bed. One parent tucks her in and gives her a kiss good-night and leaves the room.

Myths and Misconceptions

The sleep field is full of information on dos and don'ts, much of which is not based on any scientific evidence. Here are some common ones:

- No TV before bed! Up there with 'your eyes going square if you sit too close', there is actually no strong evidence to suggest watching television before bed can negatively impact young people's sleep. Of course, there are some exceptions to this. TV that could be overly stimulating should be avoided, including shows that may make your child scared, very upset or even over-excited. We should also note that there are guidelines available around screen-time for children aged 5 to 18 years (e.g. American Academy of Pediatrics), including not having a TV in the child's bedroom and not watching TV in the hour before bedtime. There are therefore other reasons you may not want your young child sitting in front of the television for a long time. However, the impact of screen-time on sleep for children is an area that needs further research before any strong conclusions can be made.

• Screen light from tablets, laptops and phones. This is one that is most relevant for older children. We know it can be a constant struggle to get kids (and most adults!) off the wide range of technologies now found in most homes. The humble mobile phone is a device that is not used just for calling and texting – it's how kids game, access the Internet, and each other ... among many other uses. In relation to sleep specifically, a key concern around the use of technologies like mobile phones and tablets or laptops is that they emit blue light, which can make you feel more alert. Common sense would say that if it were alerting then it might make it harder to fall asleep. However, there have been several studies that have tested this and most do not find that even an hour of bright screen light significantly affects sleep, at least for adolescents. A recent meta-analysis (a type of research that pools together all of the studies in the area, to draw stronger conclusions), found that the use of technology (not including television) was *slightly* related to delayed (later) sleep. But it's hard to say whether one *causes* the other – perhaps people with delayed sleep are more likely to use technology while they're awake, or perhaps the technology is responsible for delaying their sleep. It is also worth noting that much of this research is also focused on adolescents and young adults and not on younger children. Either way, to be on the safe side many technologies (e.g. mobile phones) now enable you to remove the blue light from the screen or dim the screen (for example, 'Night

Shift', found in the Display and Brightness settings on iPhones). Again, any technology that is interactive or overly stimulating should be avoided before bed, and certainly shouldn't be used in bed. Of course, there are many concerns around the use by children and teens of technology, particularly social media, and the fact that they might not be able to 'switch off' from any friendship difficulties they may face at school. Therefore, while there may be little evidence that the light from these technologies might keep your child awake, there may be other very sensible reasons not to allow your child access to these technologies in the lead-up to bed.

- Natural oils. There is little or no evidence to support most complementary or alternative treatments, outside of a placebo effect. We often find that lots of parents go through a range of these alternative treatments before they end up at our clinic. Of course, if the use of a natural oil (most commonly lavender) works for you and your child, then there is not necessarily a problem with continuing this routine. However, this doesn't target the core of their anxiety or reason for their sleep problem and is unlikely to be a long-term solution.

- Activity-monitoring watches/apps to measure sleep. With the rise of mobile apps and activity-monitoring watches, many people believe they can measure their sleep and use this as a way to establish whether they are getting enough sleep. However, research shows that these devices are not particularly accurate. They only base sleep estimates on movement, so if you move enough it will presume you are awake, or if you're lying still it will presume you are asleep. Most evidence suggests these devices are not sensitive enough and can overestimate your Total Sleep Time (TST) – making it seem like you're getting more sleep than you actually are. Also remember in Part I we talked about how the amount of sleep your child gets isn't always the same as the amount they *need*. Moreover, clock-checking behaviour (constantly looking at the time) is also often counterproductive for sleep, so keeping your phone under your pillow, where it's easily accessible, can just create more barriers to sleep.

- <u>You can 'burn' your kid's energy to get them to fall asleep</u>. Sleep pressure is important for sleep. Sometimes, parents might try to burn up their child's energy to try to get them to sleep (e.g. by getting them to race around the back garden after school, or putting them in lots of after-school activities). This might work sometimes but is not a good solution in the long run, as it doesn't tackle the reason for your child's sleep problem. It's also unlikely to help if the issue is around your child being put to bed before their body is ready to sleep, or if it is about their anxiety around being separate from a parent at night-time.

Using a Sleep Diary

All sleep intervention programmes for children need to be tailored to the needs of the individual child. Therefore, before starting any programme, it is very important to have a clear understanding of the current sleep patterns of your child. To do this, in the week before you start the programme, you should fill in a sleep diary that captures your child's *typical week* of sleep. From this sleep diary you will be able to estimate the average amount of time it takes your child to fall asleep, the average amount of sleep they are getting per night, the average time they wake up, as well as their overall sleep patterns (e.g. if / when they nap).

Completing a daily sleep diary is a good activity to do with your child so they can feel involved in the process. Completing this each morning over breakfast is the best idea. Of course, for many families with school-aged children, sitting down and eating breakfast together may be a distant memory! But do try to complete the sleep diary each day, rather than waiting and trying to complete it all at the end of the week. During a busy week, it can be difficult to accurately judge and remember the week's sleep. You may also want to record their night-time activity before you go to bed each night. However, don't let your child fill this out at night-time – we don't want the sleep diary to add to their anxiety about what time they might fall asleep.

When you are completing the sleep diary it is just an *estimate*. Again, we don't want you or your child constantly monitoring the clock as they try to fall asleep, nor when they wake during the night.

We provide some examples of sleep diaries throughout the book, and a blank copy at the back of the book that you can photocopy and use to record your own child's sleep. We use sleep diaries with all children who come through the clinic. Before we start any intervention, we get a 7-day sleep diary that shows a 'typical' week for the child's sleep. We know at first they can look confusing, so we'll take you through it step by step. At the top of the sleep diary you'll see the acronyms and definitions for key parts of your child's sleep that we introduced at the very beginning of the book.

7-day Sleep/Wake Diary

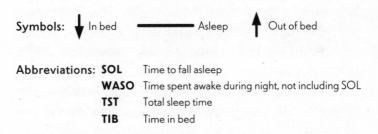

Symbols: ↓ In bed   ———— Asleep   ↑ Out of bed

Abbreviations: **SOL**   Time to fall asleep
                WASO Time spent awake during night, not including SOL
                TST   Total sleep time
                TIB   Time in bed

The meaning of each of these acronyms can be seen above under 'Abbreviations' – and remember that we have also provided these definitions at the beginning of the book (and have placed a quick description below).

To complete the sleep diary you:

1. draw downward arrows to show when they go to bed (or when you put them to bed),

2. straight horizontal lines to represent when they're asleep, and

3. use upward arrows to show when they get out of bed.

The sleep diary starts at 9 a.m., and each day is represented for the full 24 hours. If your child sleeps in after 9 a.m., the line simply continues to the next day on the following row. Below we give an example of this. You'll see this child's sleep diary for a Friday to Sunday night. On Friday night the child goes to bed around 8 p.m. (shown by the down arrow at 8 p.m. on the 'Fri' row) and reads his book for 20 minutes, falling asleep by 8.30 p.m. (this is where the beginning of the horizontal line begins). The child stays asleep all night, and then wakes up at 7.30 a.m. (as indicated by the end of the horizontal line), and gets out of bed at 7.30 a.m. (as shown by the up arrow). On Saturday night the family are out at a party and the child goes to bed at 11.30 p.m. and falls asleep in 30 minutes. The child wakes up at 10 a.m. the next day (shown on the Sunday morning) and gets out of bed at 10.30 a.m. On Sunday night, the child goes to bed around 9 p.m., falls asleep at 9.30 p.m. and wakes up at 7.30 a.m. Again, this child does not wake during the night. More details on filling in a sleep diary are presented later when we go through some case studies.

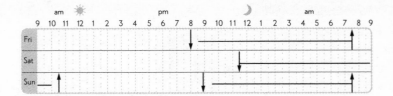

The next example of a sleep diary, recorded over two days, shows how to complete the sleep diary when your child is resisting going to bed and/or waking during the night. We'll use this example to go through how to calculate important parts of your child's sleep.

Recording how long it takes your child to fall asleep

<u>Sleep onset latency</u> (SOL) is the phrase we use for how long it takes for your child to fall asleep at the start of the night. It essentially means the 'latency' (i.e. time taken) to sleep onset (the point at which they fall asleep). We will illustrate how to record your child's sleep onset latency with the example below.

You will see that on Tuesday night this child was put to bed at 7.30 p.m. but was getting up and down until they finally fell asleep at 8.30 p.m. Her <u>sleep onset latency</u> (SOL) this night was 1 hour (i.e. it took her 1 hour to fall asleep from when she was *first* put to bed).

On Wednesday night, the child was put to bed at 8 p.m. but got up and down until 10 p.m., which means SOL was two hours.

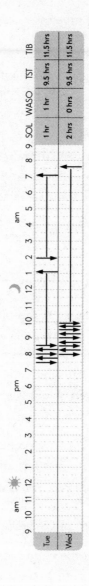

Recording how much time your child spent awake during the night

Wake After Sleep Onset (WASO) indicates how much wake time occurred after the child initially fell asleep. So WASO does not include the time in the evening when the child was put to bed – that is, it is separate from Sleep Onset Latency. This is demonstrated with the sleep diary above.

On Tuesday night, the child woke at 1 a.m. and went to their parent's bed, eventually falling back to sleep at 2 a.m. This means their wake after sleep onset (WASO) was 1 hour.

On Wednesday night, the child fell asleep at 10 p.m. and there are no significant wakings during the night, until they woke up at 7.30 a.m. and got out of bed a few minutes later. Therefore, on Wednesday night their WASO was 0 hours.

Recording how much sleep your child gets

On Tuesday night, the child fell asleep at 8.30 p.m. and woke up at 7 a.m., which is 10.5 hours. But we subtract their WASO of one hour, which means their total sleep time (TST) was 9.5 hours.

It is a bit easier to calculate the total sleep time on Wednesday night. The child fell asleep at 10 p.m. and woke at 7.30 a.m., which is 9.5 hours. Because there was no WASO during the night, then their total sleep time was the same: 9.5 hours.

Recording how much time your child spends in bed

To record your child's <u>time in bed</u> (TIB), you simply calculate the hours from when they first went to bed to when they get up out of bed. Although this child's sleep diary above shows a lot of getting into and out of bed at the start of the night, TIB nevertheless begins from the first attempt to go to bed (in this child's case that was 7.30 p.m. on Tuesday and 8 p.m. on Wednesday). On each night, this child spent 11.5 hours in bed.

Recording your child's sleep before you start the intervention

The best way to learn how to record your child's sleep is just to give it a go. We have provided you with a template for the sleep diary at the end of the book. Before you begin the intervention try to record your child's sleep for a week, to collect a 'baseline' of what a typical week of sleep looks like for your child. This is an important step for ensuring that the programme targets your child's sleep needs.

Monitoring changes in sleep

Similar to recording your child's sleep before you start any intervention, it is also important that you monitor your child's sleep throughout the programme. This is the ideal way to monitor improvements and will also tell you when you have reached their 'best' sleep routine. Keep completing the sleep diary every day each week, and at the end of the week you can look at how your child's sleep is changing – particularly any reductions in the amount of time they take to fall asleep, the number of times they get out of bed, and the amount of time they are awake during the night. This is also a great way to be able to celebrate successes with your child.

Rewards and Praise

Encouragement and praise are a great motivator for behaviour. If your child is very anxious around bedtime and will be facing this fear by trying to fall asleep without a parent present, it is important that they receive praise for this. We would encourage parents to make a sleep-chart with their child so they can celebrate successes along the way. If they fall asleep by themselves, when they wake up in the morning they can add a sticker or a stamp to their chart (combined with praise from their parent). Perhaps when they have three stamps they might get a small treat from the shops. Perhaps when they get five stamps they could be given a certificate. Looking over the improvements on the sleep diary can be a great opportunity to provide praise and encouragement. We discuss rewards and praise in more detail when we describe Exposure in Part II, chapter 5.

Setting Goals

Before starting any intervention, make sure that you are clear on what your goals are. It is best if these goals are set with your child. However, we know that sometimes the goals of parents and those of children might not match up. Your child might be perfectly happy sleeping in your bed every night! Ideally, you and your child would explore this a bit further to see if you can agree on some goals or even small steps that your child can achieve. While they may be perfectly happy sleeping in your bed, perhaps you might be able to highlight other benefits of sleeping in their own bed which may go some way to convincing them that it would be good idea. Perhaps it will help get them ready for sleepovers, or perhaps there is a new lamp or a duvet in their own room that they would get to use. Either way, it is helpful to be clear about what you want to achieve: it might be that you want to get your child falling asleep in their own bed (or on their own in your bed), your child remaining in their own bed for the whole night, or you might have another aim. But whatever your ultimate goal is, set it before you begin your programme so you are clear what you are working towards. You can write your goal(s) in the box below:

	GOAL 1	GOAL 2	GOAL 3
Example child	*Fall asleep in their own bed, without me there*	*Stay asleep in their own bed overnight*	-
Your child			

3

Helping Your Child to Fall Asleep and Stay Asleep: Bedtime and Sleep Restriction

In this chapter:

- Understanding sleep pressure (and what to do about napping)

- The sleep interventions: common questions and issues

- A step-by-step guide to Bedtime Restriction

- A step-by-step guide to Sleep Restriction

Understanding Sleep Pressure

Both of the interventions we will describe aim to work out your child's 'best' sleep time – that is, the time at which their body is ready to fall asleep, and the time it is ready to wake up. One of the reasons your child may experience difficulty falling asleep is that they are actually going to bed too early and their body is not ready to sleep. This can lead to your child lying awake – a perfect place for those anxious thoughts to creep in.

Sleep pressure is an important component of sleep, and working out when your child has built up enough sleep pressure to fall asleep is the ultimate goal of Bedtime or Sleep Restriction. In our clinical work, we use the example of a car and fuel to explain this. You might also find this a helpful way of explaining to your child why they will be 'experimenting' with a new bedtime for a while.

Imagine your child's body is a car full of fuel at the beginning of the day, and they use up this fuel during the day – at school, during after-school sport, at home. Bed is like the fuel station. Your child must use up all of their fuel before they visit the fuel station (note, we wouldn't make the same recommendation for your car!). Their sleep is the fuel, filling them back up so they have energy for the next day. Often, if your child is experiencing significant problems falling asleep, a key reason is that they haven't used up enough of their 'fuel' so aren't ready to go to the 'fuel station' – they have not built up enough sleep pressure to fall asleep.

Using Bedtime or Sleep Restriction to help your child use up more of their 'fuel' will help them fall asleep quicker. However, research shows that it also actually improves the quality of their sleep – assisting with deeper sleep and reducing periods of waking during the night (Miller et al., 2014). Therefore, a primary aim of both Bedtime Restriction and Sleep Restriction is to improve the *quality* of sleep. By building their sleep pressure and helping them fall asleep more quickly, the intervention also helps your child to *learn* that they are able to fall asleep on their own/in their own bed/ without a parent present. Perhaps, unknown to them, by building their sleep pressure and allowing them to fall asleep more quickly, they will be able to challenge the thought that bed is a place where they feel very anxious or are very unsafe.

Napping

Sleep pressure is affected by napping. If your child naps, they are topping up on 'fuel', so they'll need to then use up even more of that 'fuel' before they can go to sleep at night. Because of this, we usually say napping is a 'no-no', especially during this type of sleep intervention. Even if they are sleep deprived one night (e.g. they go to a sleepover where they don't fall asleep until midnight), we would still recommend keeping them awake the next day and not letting them nap. They should have then built up a lot of sleep pressure by night-time, and be able to fall asleep very quickly. They may be a bit grumpy for that day, but one day of grumpiness is generally preferable to falling back into poor sleeping habits.

The Sleep Interventions: Common Questions and Issues

How do I explain the new routine to my children?

Your child is likely to notice that their night-time routine will change and it is important that they are included in this process. Of course, if it was up to them they would probably be very happy to continue with the current arrangement of having Mum or Dad lie with them until they fall asleep, or being able to sleep in their parents' bed! But this doesn't mean they shouldn't have the opportunity to understand what is happening. You might use the previous example of a car visiting the fuel station to explain sleep pressure to your child. This example is especially useful to explain why they are temporarily going to bed later – it is a chance for them to feel sleepy so it is easier for them to fall asleep. If their pre-bed routine has changed, it can be useful to write this new routine out with your child so they have an idea of what the changes might be (e.g. that story time will be earlier). It might be important for siblings to be involved in this too – especially if the change in routine will impact on them too. In our clinical work we rarely find siblings get overly annoyed about their brother or sister having a temporary later bedtime. The sibling probably also does not enjoy the stress around bedtime, especially if the parent is having to focus so much energy on one child, and would like their brother or sister to be able to overcome this. Nevertheless, it is of course important to acknowledge the change of your child's bedtime to siblings. Make it clear that it is temporary and it is to help the whole family get a better and happier night-time routine. You may need to consider how your child spends their new quiet time too – their sibling may not be very happy if their brother or sister gets to watch television for an hour while they have to go to bed, but they might not care if he or she is in their room drawing. Small rewards and praise for all children for managing the new routine can also be helpful – like letting them choose their favourite dinner one night, or a movie to watch.

In this section we are going to present you with two options for sleep interventions – Bedtime Restriction and Sleep Restriction. They both follow similar patterns of temporarily moving your child's bedtime to work more effectively with sleep pressure and support them to learn to fall asleep by themselves. Either intervention is appropriate for children who experience anxiety around bedtime, including needing a parent to be with them to fall asleep, sleeping in their parent's/parents' bed, or bedtime refusal or resistance. If the main concern is that your child wakes during the night, we would generally recommend Sleep Restriction as the best approach. However, if your main concern is around their anxiety at bedtime, either intervention could be suitable.

When using Bedtime Restriction, some parents say that it takes a few nights to get into the swing of the programme. Your child may still get up and down quite a lot in the first night, until their sleep pressure builds by the middle or end of the week. Using Sleep Restriction, sleep pressure builds more quickly – because they are temporarily deprived of some sleep each night – so results usually happen very quickly.

Clinically, we find that Sleep Restriction can lead to quicker results – children tend to fall asleep very quickly, reducing anxiety fast and eliminating bedtime resistance. It can also swiftly eliminate night-time wakings. Temporarily restricting their sleep increases evening sleepiness (which is thought to dampen anxiety), and is therefore likely to reduce time awake in bed where those 'worry thoughts' might creep in. However, we also know that some parents find it tricky to manage the later bedtime that this can temporarily produce, so Bedtime Restriction might be a better option to help ensure the routine can be consistently stuck to.

The first week of the Sleep Restriction programme can be challenging. Your child may be more sleepy in the evening. However, this programme may be preferable for families who want to achieve quicker results, versus a more gradual, step-by-step approach.

Unfortunately, research is not yet advanced enough to tell us conclusively which intervention might be best. Certainly, if your child sometimes experiences parasomnias (e.g. night terrors) we would recommend that you stick with Bedtime Restriction (where their average sleep is not restricted). Our own research has shown that parasomnias are not actually negatively impacted by Bedtime or Sleep Restriction for school-aged children; however, we still need to do much more research to give conclusive advice on this. If parasomnias are not an issue, you could use either technique.

After starting the programme, what if my child still gets out of bed, even with their new bedtime?

In the first few nights of the sleep intervention (especially Bedtime Restriction), this can actually be quite common, as children are really trying to face their fears and worries. We would expect this to decrease as their sleep pressure (and sleepiness) increases. Nevertheless, it is important that you are prepared to be consistent and persistent in response to this. This might include your child getting out of bed after you have put them to bed or it might be coming into your bed during the night. In such cases we recommend you:

- Respond calmly

- Lead them back to their own bed

- Keep any conversation to an absolute minimum (avoid bargaining)

- Leave the room

- Repeat as necessary

The key to managing this issue is *persistence* and *consistency*.

The strategies we discuss in this book are the same as those we have used with many families in our clinical work. We know this isn't always easy. Everyone is tired, and parents often feel a mix of sympathy and frustration towards their child's sleep-related anxiety. Perhaps the most frustrating aspect is that parents sometimes find that their child seems to fall asleep fine with other people – when they have a babysitter or at a grandparent's house, for instance – but then are unable to when they are with their parent(s). However, we tell parents to think of this as a positive. It shows that their child can fall asleep without being over-whelmed by anxiety.

If your child gets out of bed, walk them back into their room and back into bed without fuss or conversation. Remember, it is important to avoid over-reassurance, as this can actually increase their anxiety. This means avoiding saying things like, 'It's okay, it's okay, you're safe, we checked outside, we checked the bed, we checked the wardrobe,' because this sort of reassurance might actually lead to their anxiety and alertness increasing, rather than decreasing; unintentionally it can send a message that the child does indeed have a reason to feel unsafe. Instead, lead them back to their bed, tuck them in and leave again. We know this can be a difficult step for parents as your child can become very upset that you are not staying with them. However, we usually find that after only one or two nights of parents persisting and being consistent with this process (combined with the ever-increasing sleep pressure), children's bedtime resistance dramatically (if not completely) reduces. Remember, sleep *will* eventually win over anxiety. Sometimes, we find these processes are as much about the child facing their fears as it is about parents learning that their child can indeed overcome these fears. With consistency and persistence, your child will learn that they can sleep on their own and their anxiety will reduce.

If, even after the sleep intervention, your child continues to find it difficult to sleep without you, or sleep in their own bed, they are likely to benefit from the second step of helping them face their fears step-by-step (known as Exposure), that we present later in this book (Part II, chapter 5).

My child is getting very sleepy with their later bedtime. Do I keep them awake?

Sometimes parents report that it can be challenging to actually keep their child awake until this later bedtime (especially in the first week). Persistence here is important to maintain their sleep pressure. In Sleep Restriction you are really trying to get your child to use up every last drop of their 'fuel'. Your child's sleep will only be restricted for two weeks (presuming they are falling asleep quickly and their bedtime is being moved 15 minutes earlier each week – more about that later). To try to help them stay awake they might do their quiet activity time in dim light, sitting up at a desk. Avoid letting them lie on the couch or a bean-bag where they might fall asleep. You really want them falling asleep in their own bed (if that is your goal).

Of course, if they are begging to go to their bed to fall asleep then that is great, as it means their sleepiness has definitely dampened their anxiety! In this case, they could of course go to bed. It is better that they go to bed and practise falling asleep there, rather than getting so tired that they fall asleep on the sofa during their quiet activities. If their extreme sleepiness seems to occur at the same time before bedtime every night, night after night, then this might indicate that this is the better bedtime for them.

Take note, though, whether this 'one-off' earlier bedtime during Sleep Restriction means they are awake more during the night, or even the next night. If that is the case, if you experience another night when they are asking to go to bed earlier, you may want to agree, but take your time to get them into bed so that they stay awake a bit longer and are less likely to wake up during the night.

I worked out their average total sleep and wake-up time, but it means their bedtime is very late.

This can certainly happen. We have had children ending up with quite late bedtimes for the first few weeks of these treatments, and parents can initially be quite shocked about this. First, it is important to remember that this time simply reflects the average time that they are falling asleep and so they will still be getting the same average amount of sleep that they were already getting (or slightly less with Sleep Restriction, but more on that later). What we are aiming to reduce or eliminate is their time awake, as well as their anxiety. Second, the bedtimes at the beginning of the intervention are *temporary*. Remember, short-term pain for long-term gain. Eventually, your child's bedtime will move earlier and earlier each week until you find their ideal sleep pattern.

My child refuses to fall asleep in their own bed.

Focus on changing one thing at a time – aim to get them falling asleep quickly in whichever bed they usually fall asleep in (even if it's yours). The focus should be on your child falling asleep without you present (or at least needing to lie with them). After a few nights – especially with Sleep Restriction – they may be sleepy enough to go to their own bed. If not, after finishing the sleep programme, you can move on to helping your child face their fear of sleeping in their own bed, with our step-by-step guide.

My child still takes more than 20 minutes to fall asleep, even with their later bedtime.

If this happens, simply stay on that week's sleep schedule for another week, rather than moving their bedtime 15 minutes earlier (more about that later). *Make sure you keep their wake-up time consistent, even over the weekend.* Do not let them sleep in to 'catch up' or you'll be undoing their sleep pressure. Sleep pressure should continue to build until they are falling asleep quicker. If it does not build (i.e. they are never falling asleep quicker), their sleep needs may have been slightly misjudged, so you could try moving their bedtime 15 minutes later. Once they achieve success in falling asleep quickly with the first temporary bedtime, they can then progress to the next step (moving their bedtime earlier).

As you work through the programme, each week you will move their bedtime slightly earlier. In general, after only a few weeks, you will find that your child will get to a situation where they are taking less than 20 minutes to fall asleep and then waking up well (i.e. not appearing very tired during the day). This is usually an indication that they have found their best sleep time. They have found a sleep pattern that best matches their internal 'body clock' and their sleep pressure needs. This can be later than parents would like. You may have a child that simply needs less sleep. We know it is important for parents to have their own 'wind-down' time after a busy day so, if this occurs, you do have some options. You can move their bedtime *and* wake-up time earlier. You could also move your child's quiet time to their bedroom (set up a quiet-time area there, for example). If they are worried about doing quiet time in their bedroom, you could use the steps outlined in Part II, chapter 5, where you can support them to face their worry about being in their room alone.

I'm confused about when to do story time.

Story time is part of many bedtime routines with children. Where it fits within their quiet time can depend on your child. Sometimes, it's fine to keep it just before bed, as you usually had it. So – they complete their quiet activities, then get into bed 10 minutes before bedtime, while you sit *on top of the covers* and do story time. However, where children are very anxious about separating from their parents, we've found that it can sometimes be useful to move story time to earlier in quiet time. So, as part of their quiet activities you may do their story time; then, when it's bedtime, you are only tucking them in and leaving the room. That is, you eliminate any need to sit on their bed and then have to leave again. Working out what works best for your child may just take some trial and error over the first week.

They want to sleep with their light on.

Wanting to sleep with a light on is quite common for anxious children. While we use the term 'lights out' to describe their new bedtime, this shouldn't be taken literally.

Remember to change one thing at a time. If they sleep with their light on, it's okay for them to continue this while you're doing Bedtime or Sleep Restriction. The reward of having them fall asleep by themselves and with less anxiety will usually outweigh any concern about lighting.

My child has a sleepover.

If possible, during the first two weeks of a sleep intervention, it is best to let your child focus on developing their new sleep patterns, in their own home and in their usual bed. We therefore recommend trying to keep at least two consecutive weekends free from sleepovers to give your child the best chance of success. However, if this isn't possible, then try to have the sleepover at your house so you can still have some control over your child's sleeping times. If they get less sleep on the sleepover night, still avoid letting them nap and take advantage of the extra sleep pressure to allow them to fall asleep quicker the following night. Then continue with your intervention as usual.

My child shares a room with their sibling.

In our clinical work, some children we have seen have shared a bedroom, even a bunk bed, with a sibling. In other cases, we have used one of these restriction therapies with one of two twins. These therapies can still be performed as usual; it just requires a bit more thought about how quiet the pre-bedtime activities are, as well as how dim the light should be. For example, one child had a younger sibling in the same room and they shared a bunk bed. We kept to the scheduled bedtime for the older child, and knew that the younger sibling might want to stay up as late as his brother. Our prediction was correct. However, we also predicted that the younger sibling would not be able to continue staying up later for a week – and that prediction was right as well. The younger sibling inevitably fell asleep around their usual bedtime. This allowed the older child to read with a book light and stick to the plan.

How do I fit their new sleep time around my own night-time and morning routine?

We know it's important for parents to get their own down-time before bed, so they can also have a chance to relax after their busy day. Similarly, a parent may not want to have to wake-up at 6.30 a.m. at the weekend to ensure their child is awake. Sometimes we see that parents who require a long sleep have ended up with a child who just does not need as much sleep. There is no easy answer here, and it usually just takes a bit of creativity. For mornings, you could help your child to get used to using an alarm. There are all kinds of fancy and exciting alarms available, so finding one that they love can be a great strategy. Some children particularly like how 'grown up' they feel using their alarm clock. Having activities ready that they can do when they wake up at weekends is also a good plan – so they know that when they wake up they can go and watch cartoons or keep building their Lego. If their bedtime is significantly later, it would be beneficial to encourage your child to do their quiet-time activities in their bedroom (but not in bed). You might be able to set them up a 'quiet corner' or desk in their room that is their place for quiet time. That is generally the best way we have found to manage a balance between meeting your child's sleep needs and meeting your own needs for some 'quiet time'. If they refuse to sit in their room (or feel very anxious), you could try to use the Exposure Ladder technique that we present later (Part II, chapter 5), but to move their quiet time from its current location (e.g. the kitchen table) to their bedroom. Remember, the phrase 'short-term pain for long-term gain' rings true here. A few weeks of disrupted mornings or evenings for the parent is likely worth the benefit of overcoming your child's sleep problem.

My child's wake-up time for school is 6.30 a.m. – do I now have to wake-up at 6.30 a.m. at weekends, for ever?

No. A key purpose of the intervention is to help children learn that their bed is not somewhere they need to feel scared and that they can fall asleep on their own. The consistent wake-up time is very important for the duration of the sleep intervention – usually only a few weeks. Over this time it is ideal if a parent can support the child to wake up and get moving in the morning (especially if they are doing the Sleep Restriction programme). However, in the longer term, a good part of helping your child to overcome their worries or anxiety is to let them build independence in different areas of their lives. One area might be waking up in the morning (again, perhaps supporting them to use an alarm clock). Their body clock may also simply wake them up at this time. As above, you might then have a set of activities that they can do when they wake up.

Can I do these programmes if my child experiences frequent parasomnias (like bed-wetting, night terrors, sleep-walking)?

If parasomnias are your key concern (rather than anxiety at night-time), please refer to the programme in Part III. If your concern is around bedtime anxiety/resistance/refusal, and your child happens to sometimes experience parasomnias, these programmes are still suitable to use. If your child has experienced parasomnias in the past, the Bedtime Restriction programme is unlikely to cause these parasomnias to return. Likewise, if they currently experience parasomnias, then the Bedtime Restriction techniques are unlikely to increase their frequency. Although a restriction of time in bed has meant younger children (i.e. pre-schoolers) are more likely to have parasomnias, our own research has shown that this is very rarely the case for school-aged children. However, as Sleep Restriction can exacerbate parasomnias, if your child still currently experiences parasomnias, we would suggest sticking to Bedtime Restriction.

Bedtime Restriction

Once you have been recording your child's sleep for at least a week using the sleep diary, you are ready to start the main part of the programme, where you will begin to make changes to your child's sleep schedule. We will explain two techniques. In the above Common Questions and Issues section and – briefly – below, we explain the pros and cons of each technique so that you can decide what suits you, your child, and your family best. You might wish to read through both techniques (which are similar) before making your final decision.

When Should You Use Bedtime Restriction?

If your child matches any of the following:

- Your child takes a long time to fall asleep (as a guide – more than 20 minutes)

- Your child wakes up frequently during the night

- Your child is very resistant to going to bed

- Your child is very anxious around bedtime

- Your child will only fall asleep in your bed or their sibling's bed

- Your child will only fall asleep if you stay in the room

Why Use Bedtime Restriction (Instead of Sleep Restriction)?

As discussed in the Common Questions and Issues section (pages 73–86), Bedtime Restriction is a more gentle approach as it does not involve restricting the amount of sleep that your child gets, on average. Because Sleep Restriction, as the name suggests, involves minor temporary reductions in sleep, their initial bedtime might also be too late for you to manage. If this is the case you might also prefer Bedtime Restriction. If your child experiences parasomnias (bed-wetting, night terrors), you should also stick with Bedtime Restriction.

Because it is more gentle, it might mean that – for the first few nights – your child will get up and down from bed, until they eventually fall asleep. Therefore, you should be prepared to follow the routine of putting them back to bed (see Common Questions and Issues section). If you are looking for quicker results (remember: short-term pain, long-term gain) and your child does not experience parasomnias, you might prefer Sleep Restriction, described in the next section.

What Does Bedtime Restriction Involve?

Bedtime Restriction involves shifting your child's bedtime (i.e. the time you put them to bed) to a later time, so that they have more chance of falling asleep quickly and independently and less chance of waking during the night. While keeping your child awake for even longer may seem counterproductive to many parents, it's important to remember two things. First – it should not dramatically change the amount of sleep your child is currently getting, just the amount of time they are in their bed and the *quality* of their sleep. Second – the change is only temporary, and bedtimes will continue to move until your child reaches their best bedtime.

Getting started:

Bedtime Restriction involves 4 steps:

1. Use the information from the sleep diary to work out the average amount of sleep your child is getting over the week

2. Choose a consistent wake-up time (that will suit your family and school commitments)

3. Create their new (temporary) bedtime (Step 2 minus Step 1)

4. With each week of successful sleep, move the bedtime earlier by 15 minutes, until you reach a stage where your child is falling asleep within 20 minutes and not experiencing significant daytime problems (e.g. falling asleep in class, difficulty concentrating, etc.)

The Bedtime Restriction Programme

Week 1

Establishing your child's 'new' bedtime

Once you have completed one week of the sleep diary, you need to work out:

1. The average amount of sleep they get each night (add up the amount of sleep they get each night over the week and divide it by the number of nights).

2. A consistent wake-up time that suits your child and your family (that is, the time your child needs to wake up to get everyone out the door to school on time).

Once you have set their wake-up time, you simply subtract the number of hours of sleep they receive on average. This then becomes their temporary bedtime.

In the example box below, if a child was getting an average of 9 hours' sleep per night and their wake-up time was set for 7 a.m., the first step for their new sleep schedule would be a bedtime of 10 p.m. This new, later bedtime should give them more time to build up that all-important sleep pressure. As mentioned earlier, sleep pressure helps to dampen anxiety, so by building up your child's sleep pressure you're also hopefully helping to reduce some of their night-time worries. In some cases, this first step results in the new, temporary bedtime being quite a lot later than it was. We've had cases where we end up with 7 year olds going to bed at 11 p.m. However, it is important to remember that this technique is not meant to reduce the average amount of sleep your child is already getting. Rather it is condensing the time they are in bed so that time in bed = time asleep. It is also important to remember that it is temporary.

There is space in the box below for you to enter your child's wake-up time, the average hours of sleep they got, and then their new bedtime.

	New wake–up time	Average amount of sleep	New bedtime
Example child	7 a.m.	9 hours	10 p.m.
Your child			

Note: if your child's average sleep for the week is a strange number (e.g. 9.7 hours) round it down to the nearest half-hour (e.g. 9.5 hours).

Stick to your child's new bedtime routine and timing for one week. If they are falling asleep quickly each night (in under 15 minutes, as a guide – although in the first week we would expect it to be much quicker), move their bedtime 15 minutes earlier. Carry on with this for one week and, if they continue to fall asleep quickly, move it 15 minutes earlier again. This is maintained until the child is falling asleep within (approximately) 20 minutes and is not experiencing any daytime consequences that might suggest they are sleep deprived.

There is no particular day of the week that you should start this intervention. It is all about what works best for you and your family – that is, what timing works so that you can ensure you are able to stick to the new sleep schedule.

While some families may choose to start this technique on a Friday night, which allows the child a couple of days to establish the new bedtimes before going back to school, in our experience we have found it does not matter which night to start it. It's your choice. What is important is that you feel prepared and motivated to stick to the routine.

Let's go through a step-by-step example with Thomas, who you met earlier on in the book:

Example: Thomas – 10 Years Old

Thomas is a 10-year-old boy who takes a long time to fall asleep. He lives with his mother. Night-times for Thomas and his mum are typically characterised by arguments and tears until he is so exhausted that he just falls asleep – sometimes with his mum sitting on his bed. His mum has filled out a *baseline* sleep diary (you might think of it as Week 0) to measure what his sleep is currently like. Let's go through what Thomas's sleep looks like each night before starting the programme:

Monday night: Thomas's mum put him to bed at 7.30 p.m., but Thomas was getting out of bed frequently and being put back in bed, until he fell asleep at 9 p.m. Thomas then slept through the night until his mum woke him up at 6.30 a.m. His sleep onset latency (SOL) was 1.5 hours (from 7.30 p.m. to 9 p.m.). His total sleep time (TST) was 9.5 hours.

7-day Sleep/Wake Diary

Symbols: ▼ In bed   ――― Asleep   ◀ Out of bed

Abbreviations:
SOL Time to fall asleep
WASO Time spent awake during night, not including SOL
TST Total sleep time
TIB Time in bed (time from bedtime to wake-up time)

Name .... Thomas   Baseline ....

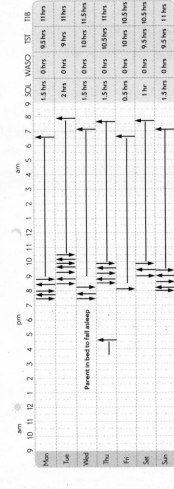

	SOL	WASO	TST	TIB
Mon	1.5 hrs	0 hrs	9.5 hrs	11 hrs
Tue	2 hrs	0 hrs	9 hrs	11 hrs
Wed	1.5 hrs	0 hrs	10 hrs	11.5 hrs
Thu	1.5 hrs	0 hrs	10.5 hrs	11 hrs
Fri	0.5 hrs	0 hrs	10 hrs	10.5 hrs
Sat	1 hr	0 hrs	9.5 hrs	10.5 hrs
Sun	1.5 hrs	0 hrs	9.5 hrs	11 hrs

Tuesday night: Thomas was put to bed later, at 8.30 p.m., and after much 'up and down', fell asleep 2 hours later at 10.30 p.m. He slept, without waking up, until approximately 7.30 a.m. His sleep onset latency (SOL) was 2 hours and his total sleep time (TST) was 9 hours.

Wednesday night: Thomas's mum was concerned that he didn't get enough sleep on Tuesday night so she put him to bed at 7.30 p.m. He got out of bed again so his mum took him back to bed and lay with him until he fell asleep. His SOL was 1.5 hours and he slept for 10 hours.

Thursday: On Thursday after school, Thomas fell asleep on the couch. As soon as his mum realised what had happened, she woke him up; she estimated he had been asleep for about 1 hour. He was then put to bed at 8.30 p.m. and was up and down until he fell asleep at 10 p.m. His SOL was 1.5 hours and his TST was 10.5 hours. Note, TST *includes* any naps.

Friday: On Friday night Thomas was put to bed at 8 p.m. and fell asleep in about 20 minutes. He slept through the night and woke up at 6.30 a.m. His mum estimated his SOL as 30 minutes and his TST as 10 hours.

Saturday: Thomas seemed to sleep quite well on Friday night (a good example of sleep pressure in action!). On Saturday night he watched a movie, so he went to bed a bit later at 9 p.m. He got up once and was eventually put back to bed, going to sleep at 10 p.m. He then slept for

9.5 hours, waking up at 7.30 a.m. His sleep onset latency was 1 hour.

Sunday: Thomas was put to bed at 8 p.m. and was up and down from bed, until he fell asleep at 9.30 p.m., making his sleep onset latency 1.5 hours. He slept through the night until he woke up at 7 a.m., after 9.5 hours of sleep.

Thomas's mum must now work out his *average* total sleep time. From the baseline sleep diary, his average total sleep time is 9.71 hours, which is rounded down to 9.5 hours.

Week 1

Thomas needs to wake up at 7 a.m. to be ready to leave for school so this becomes his consistent wake-up time. This is the time he will wake up while he is doing the Bedtime Restriction programme. The new bedtime is established by subtracting the average sleep time (9.5 hours) from the new wake-up time (7 a.m.). Thomas's new *temporary* bedtime/ lights-out time therefore becomes 9.30 p.m.[2] Thomas stays with this bedtime routine for one week.

At this first step, you may find your child's new bedtime is far later than you are currently putting them to bed. Remember – this is only temporary, and it's based on the

---

2   We often refer to bedtime as 'lights-out' time. However, some children prefer to sleep with a night-light on. 'Lights-out' time doesn't mean all the lights need to be turned off. We encourage tackling one thing at a time, so they can do the Bedtime Restriction with their usual amount of lighting.

amount of sleep they're already getting. What is being cut out is the bedtime resistance, the in-and-out-of-bed stage, the worries, and hopefully the conflict. In Part I, chapter 4 we also talked about how this later bedtime can help to dampen anxiety, or worries about sleep or their bedroom.

> *'Remember, this new bedtime is only temporary and it is based on the amount of sleep they are already getting.'*

THOMAS'S WEEK 1 SLEEP SCHEDULE:

	Quiet time	Bedtime	Wake–up time
Week 1	8.30 p.m.	9.30 p.m.	7 a.m.

You can fill in your child's week 1 schedule below:

My child's week 1 sleep schedule:

	Quiet time	Bedtime	Wake–up time
Week 1			

Managing Your Child's Pre-Bedtime Activities

If your child's bedtime becomes later, you'll need a plan for how to fill this space in the evening. Their new bedtime might now be at the same time as you usually go to bed (or sometimes even later). Therefore, it's important that this extra time is filled with activities that are a balance between your time and your child's time.

We recommend these activities begin at least an hour before bed ('quiet time') but there's no reason they couldn't start earlier. Like most things during quiet time (e.g. noise, light), your child's pre-bedtime activities should be less stimulating. And they should become quieter as they approach their new bedtime. Like using a dimmer light switch, you also want to dial down your child's pre-bedtime activities. For example, they may initially spend a bit more time in a living area watching some quiet TV in dim light, and then move to their dimly lit bedroom floor playing a quiet puzzle, or Lego, or a similar activity. Then after a while they can move to their bed (on top of their covers) for some light reading, and then under the covers to finish their reading.

Work with your child to come up with a 'menu' of activities that they can choose from. Examples might be drawing, reading, and crafts. It could also be okay to watch a relaxing movie or TV show. Remember to refer to the section on 'sleep hygiene' for 'dos and don'ts' around bedtime (Part II, chapter 2). Your child does need to stay awake during this time – as we only want them falling asleep once it is bedtime. So it's useful to make sure they're sitting up while they do these activities, rather than lying down on the couch or in a beanbag. Sitting up at the kitchen table or a desk in their room is a helpful strategy for making sure they stay awake. That said, if your child needs encouragement to be a bit sleepier at their new later bedtime, it can be okay, towards the end of their quiet/wind-down time, to get them to complete their quiet activities slouching in their bed. After all, the closer our posture is to lying down, the sleepier we feel, which is likely due to our body preparing us for sleep.

These pre-bedtime activities should be:

- A range of activities that your child can choose from

- Quiet activities (not physically or emotionally stimulating; not homework)

- Done in dim light (e.g. a lamp in your child's bedroom)

- Done for at least an hour before bedtime

Examples of activities:

- Drawing

- Craft, Lego

- Puzzles

- Reading

- Watching TV

- Listening to music

Once you have talked with your child and they have come up with their own 'menu' of different quiet activities that they can choose from each night, remember to order them so that they become less stimulating as the night goes on.

Below we have provided an example of how you can work with your child in developing a 'quiet activities menu'; at the end of the book, we've provided a blank version of this form so you can copy it and use it with your child.

QUIET ACTIVITIES MENU

Pre-bedtime activities	Quiet ratings	Quiet menu	Times
List as many activities that your child can do between dinner time and sleep time	For each activity, give it a 'quiet rating' – with 1 being very quiet and relaxing and 10 being very stimulating	List all activities that you agree are 'quiet' activities	Provide a timeframe for when the child can do each activity (between dinner and bedtime)
Playing video game (Minecraft)	9	TV	7 p.m.–8 p.m.
		LEGO	7 p.m.–8 p.m.
Watching TV in the lounge room	4	Reading	8 p.m.–9 p.m.
		Listening to music	8 p.m.–9 p.m.
Watching YouTube	8	Puzzles	8 p.m.–9 p.m.
Listening to music	1		
Playing a musical instrument	6		
Playing LEGO on the bedroom floor	3		
Reading a printed book on the bed	2		
Puzzles	4		
Jumping on the trampoline	10		

In the above example, the child can watch TV and play with their Lego before 8 p.m. (when their younger sibling then goes to bed). Then in the hour before bed he has three activities that he can choose between (reading, listening to music, puzzles).

Let's have a look at how Thomas got on in his Week 1 of Bedtime Restriction:

Thomas has completed Week 1 of Bedtime Restriction.

The first night was still difficult. He was up and down a few times and became very upset. His mother persevered with managing this via the techniques described in the earlier section. Each time he got out of bed she walked him back, gave him a kiss goodnight, said 'See you in the morning' and left his room. He was becoming quite upset by this but she persevered and by 10.30 p.m. he fell asleep.

The second night he only got out of bed once after bedtime, and his mum again stuck to their routine.

After only two nights, Thomas was falling asleep at his new temporary bedtime and staying asleep.

Thomas was sleeping through the night. He also said that he wasn't waking up as much during the night and didn't feel as if he was having as many bad dreams (which can be a child's way of saying they feel less anxious). This may seem like an almost impossible improvement, but we have seen it over and over again in our clinical work.

7-day Sleep/Wake Diary

Symbols: ↓ In bed   ——— Asleep   ↑ Out of bed

Abbreviations: **SOL**   Time to fall asleep
                WASO Time spent awake during night, not including SOL
                TST   Total sleep time
                TIB   Time in bed (time from bedtime to wake-up time)

Name .... *Thomas* ....   **Week 1 Bedtime Restriction Therapy**

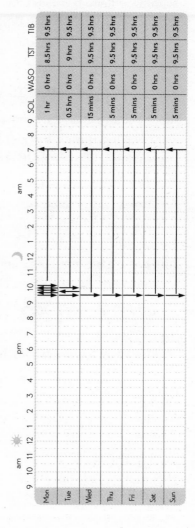

	SOL	WASO	TST	TIB
Mon	1 hr	0 hrs	8.5 hrs	9.5 hrs
Tue	0.5 hrs	0 hrs	9 hrs	9.5 hrs
Wed	15 mins	0 hrs	9.5 hrs	9.5 hrs
Thu	5 mins	0 hrs	9.5 hrs	9.5 hrs
Fri	5 mins	0 hrs	9.5 hrs	9.5 hrs
Sat	5 mins	0 hrs	9.5 hrs	9.5 hrs
Sun	5 mins	0 hrs	9.5 hrs	9.5 hrs

Thomas is falling asleep very quickly and seems sleepier when he is woken (i.e. harder to wake up). Therefore, he is ready to move on to Week 2 – and so are you!

Week 2

After one week of your child's temporary bedtime you should notice that they are falling asleep faster. If they were waking during the night, you may notice that they are waking less (perhaps there are fewer nights on which they come into your room, for instance).

Sometimes it can take a while to adjust to this new routine. Your child may be a little more tired during the day, especially towards the end of the week. However, it is important to persevere and stick to your Week 1 schedule.

At the end of Week 1, if you notice your child is falling asleep quickly, and there's been less anxiety or resistance, then you can move on to the Week 2 treatment plan.

If your child is taking a bit longer to settle into their new routine, stick to Week 1's plan for one more week.

If your child is still finding it very difficult to fall asleep, you may have misjudged their original sleep timing. Try making their bedtime 15 minutes later for the next week. Eventually, their sleep pressure will build up and help them fall asleep more easily.

Now let's see how Thomas is getting on . . .

- His bedtime moves 15 minutes earlier (because Thomas is taking less than 20 minutes to fall asleep in Week 1)

- Thomas's wake-up time stays at the same time

Thomas's week 2 sleep schedule:

	Quiet time	Bedtime	Wake-up time
Week 2	8.15 p.m.	9.15 p.m.	7 a.m.

Thomas's new bedtime in Week 2 is now 9.15 p.m., making his quiet time from 8.15 p.m. His wake-up time stays at 7 a.m.

You can fill in your child's Week 2 schedule below:

My child's week 2 sleep schedule:

	Quiet time	Bedtime	Wake-up time
Week 2			

From his Week 2 sleep diary you can see that Thomas is now falling asleep quickly most nights. On the Saturday

7-day Sleep/Wake Diary

Symbols: ↓ In bed   ━━ Asleep   ← Out of bed

Abbreviations:
SOL Time to fall asleep
WASO Time spent awake during night, not including SOL
TST Total sleep time
TIB Time in bed (time from bedtime to wake-up time)

Name ...... Thomas ......   Week 2 Bedtime Restriction

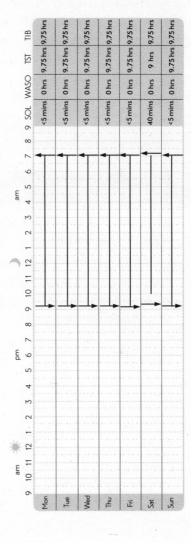

	SOL	WASO	TST	TIB
Mon	<5 mins	0 hrs	9.75 hrs	9.75 hrs
Tue	<5 mins	0 hrs	9.75 hrs	9.75 hrs
Wed	<5 mins	0 hrs	9.75 hrs	9.75 hrs
Thu	<5 mins	0 hrs	9.75 hrs	9.75 hrs
Fri	<5 mins	0 hrs	9.75 hrs	9.75 hrs
Sat	40 mins	0 hrs	9 hrs	9.75 hrs
Sun	<5 mins	0 hrs	9.75 hrs	9.75 hrs

night, Thomas had a busy day and found it a bit trickier to settle down. However, you can see that he still managed to stay in his own bed. Thomas's mum has stuck very consistently to the wake-up time, allowing Thomas to build up the necessary sleep pressure during the day. Because he's still falling asleep quickly, he can now move to a third week of Bedtime Restriction.

Week 3

By the end of Week 2, you should notice your child falling asleep quite quickly (in under 15–20 minutes) and sleeping more through the night. Remember to complete the full week at this new bedtime, and then, if your child is still falling asleep quickly (like Thomas), move to Week 3. If your child is still taking more than 20 minutes to fall asleep in Week 2, stick to this same Week 2 schedule for one more week before moving on.

Thomas's week 3 sleep schedule:

	Quiet time	Bedtime	Wake–up time
Week 3	8 p.m.	9 p.m.	7 a.m.

Thomas's new bedtime in Week 3 is now 9 p.m., making his quiet time from 8 p.m. His wake-up time stays at 7 a.m. Now he will be getting an opportunity to sleep at night for approximately 10 hours.

Remember to complete the schedule for your child too:

My child's week 3 sleep schedule:

	Quiet time	Bedtime	Wake-up time
Week 3			

You can see from Thomas's sleep diary that he is now taking approximately 15 minutes to fall asleep each night. His mum also reports that he does not appear sleepy during the day. This suggests that Thomas has discovered his 'best' bedtime. Therefore, this becomes Thomas's new sleep routine.

If 9 p.m. is too late, Thomas's mum might decide to make his bedtime 8.30 p.m. and his wake-up time 6.30 a.m. Or she may be happy with him going to bed at 9 p.m. if he sits in his room for quiet time from 8 p.m. Remember – how much sleep your child needs is unique to them. If they wake up relatively easily and function well during the day, it probably means they're having enough sleep, even if it's a little less or more than their peers are getting (or their parents want!).

7-day Sleep/Wake Diary

Symbols: ▼ In bed   ▬▬▬ Asleep   ◀ Out of bed

Abbreviations: **SOL**   Time to fall asleep
                WASO   Time spent awake during night, not including SOL
                TST   Total sleep time
                TIB   Time in bed (time from bedtime to wake-up time)

Name   *Thomas*

Week 3 Bedtime Restriction

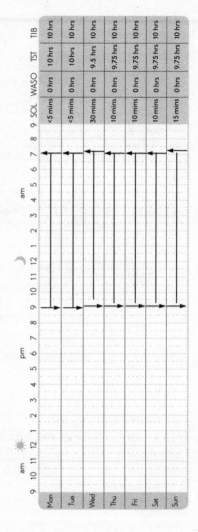

	SOL	WASO	TST	TIB
Mon	<5 mins	0 hrs	10 hrs	10 hrs
Tue	<5 mins	0 hrs	10 hrs	10 hrs
Wed	30 mins	0 hrs	9.5 hrs	10 hrs
Thu	10 mins	0 hrs	9.75 hrs	10 hrs
Fri	10 mins	0 hrs	9.75 hrs	10 hrs
Sat	10 mins	0 hrs	9.75 hrs	10 hrs
Sun	15 mins	0 hrs	9.75 hrs	10 hrs

Your Turn...

Below we have provided a Weekly Schedule that you can complete for your child. We have also provided the same table at the back of this book if you wish to copy it on to a separate piece of paper and fill it out.

My Child's Bedtime Restriction Schedule

Bedtime Restriction with a child who does not sleep in their own bed

So far we have taken you through how to do Bedtime Restriction with 10-year-old Thomas – who had difficulty sleeping in his own bed – as well as teaching you how to do Bedtime Restriction with your own child.

If you felt that Thomas's example did not match your own child's situation – for example, that your child has trouble sleeping and is in your own bedroom – or that you want to read about another example of using Bedtime Restriction before you undertake it with your own child, then please continue reading.

If you feel ready to do Bedtime Restriction with your own child, you are welcome to begin. However, we would suggest that you first read about the alternative technique called Sleep Restriction. While Bedtime Restriction and Sleep Restriction are very similar, reading about both techniques can nevertheless help you make a better decision as to which technique best suits your child. Remember, you can find the 'pros and cons' of Bedtime v. Sleep Restriction in the earlier Common Questions and Issues section (page 87).

	Quiet time	Bedtime	Wake-up time
Week 1 Date			
Week 2 Date			
Week 3 Date			

Example: Sophie – 6 Years Old

Unlike Thomas, Sophie needs a parent to lie down with her to fall asleep at the start of the night in her bedroom, yet Sophie spends most nights sleeping in her parents' bed, or on a mattress in their room. She would be happy to fall asleep in her own bed if her mum was in the bed with her, but this was becoming practically difficult because of the size of Sophie's bed (besides the fact that her mum would like her own space!). Sophie also shares a room with her younger brother, who was getting woken up with all the fuss around bedtime. If Sophie falls asleep in her parents' bed, she will sometimes get moved back to her bed. However, she will then often wake up at night and move back to her parents' room. At the moment, to try to ensure everyone can sleep, Sophie's parents have set up a mattress in their room where Sophie can sleep. Despite the different – and perhaps more complex – presentation, compared to Thomas, Sophie's Bedtime Restriction programme will still follow the same pattern we described for Thomas. In clinical practice, we sometimes find that the later bedtime means children are sleepy enough to fall asleep in their own bed from the beginning of treatment (especially if you choose to do Sleep Restriction, which we present in the next section). However, if this is not the case, remember the tip is to change one thing at a time. So Sophie may start her treatment falling asleep in her parents' bed (with the goal being that she falls asleep in their bed but without them with her). Or she may start it back in her own bed but with her parent standing by the doorway (but not in the bed with her). Her parents can then use 'exposure' to support Sophie to face her worries and sleep in her own bed.

Sophie's sleep

From Sophie's *baseline* sleep diary (page 112) we can work out that it takes her an average of just over 1 hour to fall asleep each night (1 hour SOL). She also gets an average of just under 9.5 hours' total sleep time (TST) each night (her wake-up times are not included). Let's go through each night of Sophie's baseline:

Monday: Sophie's parent put her to bed in her own bed around 7.30 p.m. but then she is up and down many times until her mum sits with her and she eventually falls asleep at

9 p.m. (1.5 hours SOL). She stays asleep in her own bed until she wakes up at approximately 2.30 a.m. and comes into her parents' room and sleeps on the spare mattress for the rest of the night. She is woken up at 7 a.m. and gets out of bed at 7.30 a.m.

Tuesday: Sophie is put into her own bed at 8 p.m. but gets up almost straight away and is very upset. Her brother was also woken up, so her parents put her in their bed and she falls asleep by around 8.30 p.m. (0.5 hour SOL). She wakes up at 7 a.m.

Wednesday: On Wednesday night Sophie's parents decide that they will try to focus on taking her back to her own bed. She is put to bed at 8 p.m., but is up and down frequently. However, Sophie's parents take turns taking her back to her own bed every time. Sophie eventually falls asleep at 9.30 p.m. (1.5 hour SOL). She wakes up around 11.30 p.m., and while they try to take her back to her bed, they don't want to wake up her brother and she ends up sleeping in their room from 12.30 a.m. She wakes up briefly again at 5.30 a.m., but settles after 30 minutes.

Thursday: Sophie is put to bed at 8 p.m. but gets up almost immediately. Her parents put her back to bed in their room and her mum lies with her until she falls asleep. Even with her mum there, it takes her another 1.5 hours to fall asleep (total SOL 2 hours).

Friday: Friday evening is a slightly later night and Sophie isn't put to bed until 9 p.m. Her parents put her to bed in their room on her mattress. She gets up once and then her dad lies with her and she falls asleep (0.5 hour SOL). She then wakes for the day at 7 a.m.

Saturday: Saturday evening is a good example of sleep pressure. Friends are over for dinner and Sophie does not go to bed until 10.30 p.m. She falls asleep in her own bed and stays asleep all night until 7 a.m.

Sunday: Sophie is put to bed around 8 p.m. She gets up and down a few times. Her parents know she had a late night on Saturday and has school tomorrow, so they put her into their bedroom and she sleeps there, with one 30-minute Wake After Sleep Onset (WASO) around 3.30 a.m. She is then woken up for school at 7 a.m.

Sophie is taking an average of 1 hour to fall asleep each night (1 hour SOL) and sleeps for an average of 9.5 hours. While she is currently sleeping until around 7.30 a.m. on weekdays, Sophie actually needs to wake up by 6.30 a.m. so the family can get to school on time. So 6.30 a.m. becomes her *consistent wake-up time*. This is the time Sophie will have to wake up every morning over her sleep interventions, including the weekends. Sophie already has an alarm clock that she enjoys using, so they will set this so she is now woken at 6.30 a.m.

7-day Sleep/Wake Diary

Symbols: ↓ In bed   ── Asleep   ◄ Out of bed

Abbreviations:
SOL   Time to fall asleep
WASO Time spent awake during night, not including SOL
TST   Total sleep time
TIB   Time in bed (time from bedtime to wake-up time)

Name .... *Sophie* ....   Baseline

	9	10	11	12	1	2	3	4	5	6	7	8	9	10	11	12	1	2	3	4	5	6	7	8	9	SOL	WASO	TST	TIB
Mon							Parents' bed from 3am																			1.5 hrs	0.5 hrs	9.5 hrs	12 hrs
Tue							Parents' bed all night																			0.5 hrs	0 hrs	11 hrs	11.5 hrs
Wed							Parents' room from 12.30pm																			1.5 hrs	1.5 hrs	8.5 hrs	11.5 hrs
Thu							Parents' room all night																			2 hrs	0.5 hrs	9 hrs	11.5 hrs
Fri							Parents' room all night																			0.5 hrs	0.5 hrs	9.5 hrs	10.5 hrs
Sat																										0 hrs	0 hrs	9.5 hrs	9.5 hrs
Sun							Parents' bed all night																			2 hrs	0.5 hrs	9.5 hrs	12 hrs

Sophie's bedtime routine

Before beginning the programme, Sophie's parents plan her bedtime routine to ensure she has the best chance of falling asleep. Sophie will continue to have the night-light on in her room (which her brother also wants). At 7 p.m. Sophie has a short shower, brushes her teeth and gets in her pyjamas. By around 7.30 p.m., Sophie and one of her parents start to read a book together on the sofa. Sometimes this also creeps into the beginning of her quiet time, which is fine as it's a relaxing activity. At the beginning of quiet time, Sophie's parents check whether she needs the toilet and she has a final small drink before bed.

When it gets to Sophie's new bedtime, one parent takes her to bed, she is tucked in, given a kiss goodnight and then they leave the room. Sophie is able to choose to go to sleep in her parents' bedroom but the routine remains the same (i.e. they do not stay with her).

Week 1

Sophie's new temporary bedtime for Week 1 will be 9 p.m. (9.5 hours before her wake-up time of 6.30 a.m.). Because Sophie was spending most nights in her parents' bed, including with a parent lying with her, she begins her programme falling asleep *on her own* in her parents' bed. Her quiet time starts by at least 8 p.m. During her quiet/ wind-down time Sophie does some drawing and quiet craft under dim light. Because her younger brother is already in bed at this time, Sophie's quiet activity happens around the kitchen table.

Sophie's week 1 sleep schedule:

	Quiet time	Bedtime	Wake–up time
Week 1	8 p.m.	9 p.m.	6.30 a.m.

The first night was difficult for Sophie's parents. When they left their bedroom, Sophie became very upset. She got off the mattress on her parents' bedroom floor, but they followed the plan and calmly led her back to their room. This happened around ten times and lasted for 30 minutes (although it felt like much longer for her parents), but she eventually fell asleep on her own. By the second night, Sophie was falling asleep on the mattress in her parents' bedroom without her mum or dad needing to lie down with her (as Sophie was sleepy enough to fall asleep on her own). Her parents have particularly noticed a big change in Sophie's sleep at night-time (i.e. her *sleep quality*). Previously, because Sophie had often been so anxious around bed, her sleep seemed to be very light and disrupted (she would move around a lot and wake up relatively frequently). Within the first week, her night-time wakings have been almost completely eliminated, and her parents report that Sophie is getting better-quality sleep. When Sophie's parents go to bed, they are now gently moving her back to her own bed where she is staying asleep all night, with the exception of Thursday night, when she came back into their room at 5.30 a.m.

7-day Sleep/Wake Diary

Symbols: ▼ In bed   ▬▬▬ Asleep   ◀— Out of bed

Abbreviations: **SOL**   Time to fall asleep
               WASO   Time spent awake during night, not including SOL
               TST   Total sleep time
               TIB   Time in bed (time from bedtime to wake-up time)

Name   *Sophie*   Week 1 Bedtime Restriction Therapy

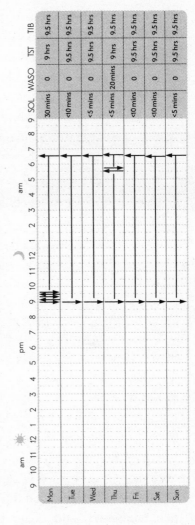

	SOL	WASO	TST	TIB
Mon	30 mins	0	9 hrs	9.5 hrs
Tue	<10 mins	0	9.5 hrs	9.5 hrs
Wed	<5 mins	0	9.5 hrs	9.5 hrs
Thu	<5 mins	20 mins	9 hrs	9.5 hrs
Fri	<10 mins	0	9.5 hrs	9.5 hrs
Sat	<10 mins	0	9.5 hrs	9.5 hrs
Sun	<5 mins	0	9.5 hrs	9.5 hrs

Week 2

As Sophie has fallen asleep quickly for most of the week, her Week 2 programme sees her bedtime move 15 minutes earlier. For Week 2 her bedtime is moved to 8.45 p.m., with quiet time from at least 7.45 p.m. (although it's usually started a bit earlier when her younger brother is put to bed). Remember, if *your* child is still taking a while to fall asleep or waking during the night, stick with your Week 1 plan for one more week before moving on.

Sophie's week 2 sleep schedule

	Quiet time	Bedtime	Wake–up time
Week 2	7.45 p.m.	8.45 p.m.	6.30 a.m.

Sophie is now falling asleep on her own. On Monday and Tuesday night she actually fell asleep and stayed asleep in her own bed. Wednesday to Friday night she slept on the mattress, but still fell asleep by herself. On Saturday Sophie's family had friends over so she was put to bed at 9.30 p.m. Because this meant her sleep pressure built up even more it is perhaps unsurprising that she was able to fall asleep in her own bed this night. Sticking to their routine, Sophie was still woken up at her standard wake-up time of 6.30 a.m. and then fell asleep very quickly on Sunday night. You'll notice Sophie's time asleep matches her time in bed – this is exactly what we are aiming for.

7-day Sleep/Wake Diary

Symbols: ↓ In bed   ——— Asleep   ◀— Out of bed

Abbreviations:
SOL Time to fall asleep
WASO Time spent awake during night, not including SOL
TST Total sleep time
TIB Time in bed (time from bedtime to wake-up time)

Name *Sophie* **Week 2 Bedtime Restriction Therapy**

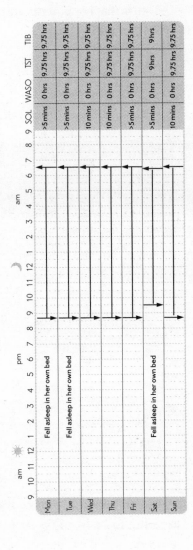

	SOL	WASO	TST	TIB
Mon	>5 mins	0 hrs	9.75 hrs	9.75 hrs
Tue	>5 mins	0 hrs	9.75 hrs	9.75 hrs
Wed	10 mins	0 hrs	9.75 hrs	9.75 hrs
Thu	10 mins	0 hrs	9.75 hrs	9.75 hrs
Fri	>5 mins	0 hrs	9.75 hrs	9.75 hrs
Sat	>5 mins	0 hrs	9 hrs	9 hrs
Sun	10 mins	0 hrs	9.75 hrs	9.75 hrs

Mon: Fell asleep in her own bed
Tue: Fell asleep in her own bed
Sat: Fell asleep in her own bed

One of the key reasons that Sophie's intervention is going so well is that her parents are adhering strictly to the agreed wake-up time.

> *'One of the key reasons that Sophie's intervention is going so well is that her parents are adhering strictly to the agreed wake-up time.'*

After two weeks of the intervention, Sophie is now able to fall asleep by herself. On three nights she even fell asleep in her own bed. The other nights she was able to fall asleep in her parents' bedroom and they did not have to lie down with her. Sophie is still falling asleep very quickly and, therefore, for the third week, they move her bedtime to 8.30 p.m., with quiet time from 7.30 p.m. Her wake-up time remains at 6.30 a.m.

Sophie's week 3 sleep schedule:

	Quiet time	Bedtime	Wake-up time
Week 3	7.30 p.m.	8.30 p.m.	6.30 a.m.

With this bedtime, Sophie reaches her ideal routine. She is going to bed at 8.30 p.m., taking about 10 minutes to fall asleep and is waking up easily in the morning. She no longer wakes for significant periods of time during the night. There are no concerns that she is more tired

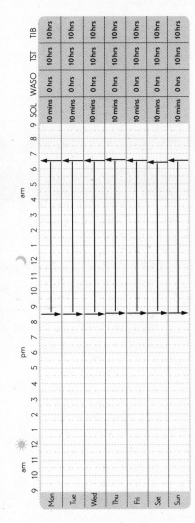

than usual during the day. She is getting 10 hours of sleep per night, which means her total sleep time has actually increased during the intervention.

What Next?

In many cases the 3-week sleep programme (like with 10-year-old Thomas) is enough to get your child's sleep back on track. However, if your child's sleep patterns remain closer to Sophie's – they might still be sleeping in your bed, or need you in their room to fall asleep – go to Part II, chapter 5, for the description of Exposure, a step-by-step guide to help your child to face their anxiety and become more confident about sleeping in their own room.

If you find that Bedtime Restriction helped your child to fall asleep quicker, but they are still waking up for a significant amount of time during the night (e.g. more than 20 minutes), and/or move from their bedroom to your bedroom during the middle of the night, you can try Sleep Restriction. If you find that Sleep Restriction does not resolve your child's wakefulness during the night, then move on to Exposure.

Sleep Restriction

When Should You Use Sleep Restriction?

As with Bedtime Restriction, this programme is suitable if your child matches any of the following:

- Your child takes a long time to fall asleep

- Your child wakes up frequently during the night

- Your child is very resistant to going to bed

- Your child is very anxious around bedtime

- Your child will only fall asleep in your bed or their sibling's bed

- Your child will only fall asleep if you stay in the room

AND

- Your main concern is <u>not</u> parasomnias (e.g. night terrors, sleepwalking: see Part III)

What Does Sleep Restriction Involve?

With the goal of having the child falling asleep by themselves and in their own bed, in our clinical experience, Sleep Restriction often only takes 2 weeks. The intervention follows the same pattern as Bedtime Restriction; however, as the name suggests, the first step involves temporarily restricting your child's sleep by 30 minutes. Sleep Restriction has been used as a treatment for adult insomnia since 1987 (Spielman et al., 1987). Over the past few years in our clinical work we have been adapting and trialling this treatment for children. In a recent study we used Sleep Restriction with over 50 families and have found substantial improvements both in the time it takes them to fall asleep and in their night-time anxiety.

A Sleep Restriction plan is worked out in a very similar way to Bedtime Restriction, but bedtime is then moved *half an hour later in the first week*. That is, from the sleep diary, work out your child's average amount of sleep each night and also the time you want them to wake up each morning. From here you will be able to work out their new bedtime, as you would for Bedtime Restriction. But what makes Sleep Restriction different is that you make the new bedtime even later, by 30 minutes. This means each night (for the first week) they are getting 30 minutes less sleep than their usual average amount of sleep.

Sleep Restriction involves 5 steps:

1. Use the sleep diary to work out the average amount of sleep your child is getting over the week

2. Choose a consistent wake-up time (that will suit your family and school commitments)

3. Create a temporary bedtime (Step 2 minus Step 1)

4. Now make bedtime 30 minutes later (Step 3 + 30 minutes). This is their new bedtime

5. With each week of successful sleep, move the bedtime earlier, until you reach a stage where your child is falling asleep within 20 minutes and not experiencing significant daytime problems (e.g., falling asleep in class, difficulty concentrating, etc.)

Because your child is going to be a bit sleep restricted, it might be a good idea to let their teacher know that you're working through this programme for the next few weeks. Overall, in our clinical work, we find that many children are quite robust in the face of short-term sleep deprivation, and teachers rarely notice a large difference. Our research has also shown that Sleep Restriction does not change children's performance on cognitive tests. Nevertheless, it might be best to inform their teacher, just in case the teacher sees any other change in your child.

As with Bedtime Restriction, their bedtime should be moved earlier each week until reaching their optimum bedtime. In Bedtime Restriction you will remember we moved bedtime 15 minutes earlier each week. In Sleep Restriction, because we expect quicker results, after the first week of restriction, you might decide to move their bedtime 30 minutes earlier for Week 2.

How Do I Decide by How Much to Move Their Bedtime in Sleep Restriction?

In our clinical work, this is what we use as a general guide:

- In Week 1, their bedtime should be restricted by 30 minutes each night, for the full week

- During Week 1, if they are falling asleep immediately and are getting tired during the day, you may wish to move their bedtime 30 minutes earlier for Week 2

- If they are still taking some time to fall asleep and don't seem to be very tired during the day, you could stick with moving it 15 minutes each week, until you reach their best bedtime

Sophie, 6 Years Old

In the case of Sophie, although Bedtime Restriction allowed her to fall asleep by herself, she was still mostly needing to fall asleep in her parents' bedroom. It then took the additional weeks of the plan to reach the ultimate goal of Sophie falling asleep in her own bed, without a parent needing to be present (described in Part II, chapter 5). For Sophie, Sleep Restriction (instead of Bedtime Restriction) might have been a better way of getting her back to sleep in her own bed earlier on.

What would her Sleep Restriction plan look like?

Week 1

Sophie's set wake-up time was 6.30 a.m. Before she started the intervention, her parents worked out that she was getting an average of around 9.5 hours' sleep each night. In the first week of sleep restriction, Sophie's sleep will be restricted to 9 hours per night. Therefore, her new bedtime for week 1 is 9.30 p.m. Her quiet time will begin at 8.30 p.m. at the latest (although quiet activities can begin earlier if necessary).

Sophie's week 1 sleep schedule:

	Quiet time	Bedtime	Wake-up time
Week 1	8.30 p.m.	9.30 p.m.	6.30 a.m.

In the first week of putting this into practice, Sophie's parents reported that by 9.30 p.m. she was extremely sleepy. While the first night saw her get up once after being put to bed, by the second night she was able to go straight to bed in her own bed and fall asleep. After only 1 week she had already made significant progress. She was waking up fine in the morning but was more tired than normal after school.

Week 2

Sophie has now had a whole week of 'practising' falling asleep by herself in her own bed. This allows her to learn that she does not need to feel scared about sleeping in her own bed. Because she is falling asleep very quickly and in her own bed, for Week 2 of Sleep Restriction her bedtime was moved to 9 p.m.

Sophie's week 2 sleep schedule

	Quiet time	Bedtime	Wake up
Week 2	8 p.m.	9 p.m.	6.30 a.m.

In Week 2, Sophie continued to fall asleep in her own bed, without needing a parent present. She was still very tired by her 9 p.m. bedtime, and there were a few nights where her parents really had to put effort into keeping her awake.

Week 3

For Week 3, Sophie's bedtime was again moved 30 minutes earlier, as she has now had 2 weeks of falling asleep in her own bed without a parent present.

Sophie's week 3 sleep schedule

	Quiet time	Bedtime	Wake-up time
Week 3	7.30 p.m.	8.30 p.m.	6.30 a.m.

Sophie has now reached her best bedtime and wake-up time and is getting approximately 10 hours' sleep per night. In this example using Sleep Restriction, you can see that her increased sleep pressure, as a consequence of her restricted sleep, meant that she was able to quickly transition back to sleeping in her own bed.

Below is the sleep schedule for you to fill out with your own child. This is the same template as was used in the Bedtime Restriction section and can also be found in the Appendix.

My child's sleep restriction schedule:

	Quiet time	Bedtime	Wake-up time
Week 1 Date			
Week 2 Date			
Week 3 Date			

Where To From Here?

At this point you are likely experiencing one of two outcomes. Either Bedtime Restriction or Sleep Restriction has been sufficient to achieve your goals (so your child now falls asleep in their own bed without you present). If that's the case, congratulations! We would still suggest you keep a close eye on your child's daytime sleepiness, to ensure they are getting enough sleep now that the programme has finished. Over the coming weeks, if they start to show consistent signs of daytime sleepiness, consider giving them a slightly earlier bedtime (e.g. 15 minutes earlier) for a week or two, and see if that helps. Although sleep pressure can build quickly over days for the benefit of your child, it can also build up over weeks and months. So you may need to change their bedtimes a bit, now and again. If your child begins to be awake a lot in bed, you may want to give them a slightly later bedtime for a week or two. Alternatively, if they become a bit sleepy, then give them an earlier bedtime for a week or two. We would also recommend that you continue reading the rest of this book. It will get you familiar with other sleep problems that can occur, and what to do about them. We even give you a sneak preview of what the sleep of a teenager can look like, and how to prepare for it.

Second, the Bedtime or Sleep Restriction programme may not have fully resolved your child's sleep problem. Some nights they might fall asleep on their own but other nights they are still continuing to get up and down and becoming very upset or frustrated. If this is happening, it is time to move on to the next technique, which involves supporting your child to overcome their fears and worries around bedtime.

4

Helping Your Child to Understand and Challenge Their Night-Time Fears and Worries

In this chapter:

- An introduction to identifying worrying thoughts

- Understanding the connection between situations, thoughts, feelings and behaviours

- How to teach your child to look for evidence and challenge their worry thoughts

- Supporting your child to problem-solve

Even if you have found either Bedtime Restriction or Sleep Restriction to be helpful, and your child has already achieved the goal of falling asleep and staying asleep in their own bed (if this was your goal), it can be useful for children (particularly older children) who are 'over-thinkers' or 'worriers' to learn how to manage and challenge their anxious thoughts. Being analytical about our own unhelpful thoughts can be a handy skill in life to have.

For younger children, where we often see lots of 'magical thinking' – *the garden gnomes are going to take me; a witch is going to come in and take Mummy* – we would usually go straight to Exposure (Part II, chapter 5), where children learn via being exposed to their fear (step by step) that their thought did not come true.

In this section we describe techniques that are known as cognitive techniques. These techniques are often central to psychological interventions for anxiety, and involve working with your child to identify what thoughts are going through their minds when they experience intense and unpleasant emotions (e.g. anxiety/fear). Cognitive techniques help children (and adults) to critically analyse these thoughts. The end result is that we begin to learn that the thoughts that make us feel very worried are not necessarily true. That is, there is a high probability that they won't happen and, if they do, the end result is not that bad.

School-aged kids have very good imaginations – but sometimes this works against them when trying to sleep by themselves at night. Children's fears and worries peak during middle childhood. Studies show that this can be primarily media-driven – that is, the things they see on the TV (e.g. crimes they see on the news), the movies they watch, and the Internet (e.g. YouTube videos) (Muris et al., 2000). We've also seen that a wave of fear occurs across schools when children begin to spread scary stories. Such stories can send children's thoughts down a scary path, and scary images can be easily recalled by children when they hear a bump in the night or when they are lying in the dark.

Linking Situations, Thoughts, Feelings and Behaviours

In this section, we will use an example that will demonstrate how situations, thoughts, feelings and behaviours are linked. It's an example we've used hundreds of times with families in our clinical and research work and demonstrates how you can work with your child's unpleasant thoughts. It may not necessarily stop the thoughts altogether, but it may help to reduce their impact.

We like to use a light-switch analogy. However, although we can turn a light off at the switch, we cannot suddenly switch off the thoughts running through our minds. Instead, it's more like a dimmer light switch. We can lower the intensity of the light by turning the knob and, likewise, we can gradually reduce the frequency and intensity of the unpleasant thoughts running through our minds.

> *'We cannot suddenly switch off the thoughts running through our minds. Instead, it's more like a dimmer light switch.'*

The Situation: Things that Go Bump in the Night

So let's start the example – beginning with the *situation*.

Imagine a child lying wide awake in their bed during the night. Suddenly, they hear a sound outside . . .

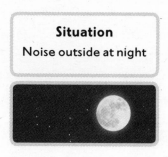

Situation
Noise outside at night

The feelings

Kids often react to a noise outside at night with an overwhelming *feeling* of being scared. This can be expressed in various ways, including a racing heart, shallow breathing, and being wide-eyed. These are all physiological reactions that we explained in Part I, chapter 4. When helping children to understand worried or scared feelings, we find a good starting place is to give the child an example and help them to work it through. This involves asking, 'If you hear a sound outside, how does that make you feel?' Most of these kids say, 'Scared', or something similar, like 'Frightened' or 'Anxious' or 'Worried'. Some children may be too shy to admit such feelings, so in these instances it is best instead to use another child in the example – so we use 'George', and thus we ask kids, 'If George heard a noise outside at night, how would he feel?'

We might then get the child to think about how they (or George) might feel in their body when they're feeling scared. Below is an example of how a child may describe how it feels in their body when they are scared (we have included a blank picture in the appendix (page 227) so you can do this activity with your child). This is an excellent activity to do with your child to help them to understand why their body feels a particular way when they are very worried. Get your child to imagine a time when they felt very worried. Or, use the example of George hearing a crash outside at night-time. Ask them – How might George feel? What might that worry feel like in their (or George's) body, working through different body parts? How does it feel in your stomach when you are anxious? Does it go around and around like a washing machine? Does it feel like little butterflies are fluttering around inside? How might it feel in their legs? Are they shaky? Or are they heavy and frozen? How might their hands feel? Hot, clammy? What about their heart? Is it beating very fast? Work through the picture to look at all the different ways their (or George's) body reacts when they feel worried. From this activity the message is – no wonder it's hard to fall asleep with all of those things going on in your body!

'No wonder it's hard to fall asleep with all of those things going on in your body!'

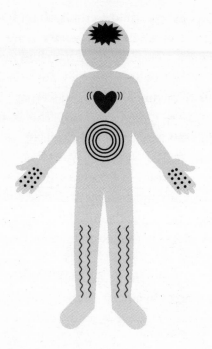

How does your body feel when you're scared?

- heart beats fast
- tummy goes round and round, like a washing machine
- palms are sweaty
- legs tremble or shake
- headache

Before the feeling . . .

Now they have labelled their feeling, and identified how that might feel in their body, we next teach them that we do not actually go straight from a *situation* to a *feeling*. As fast as this connection might feel, there is something that happens in between – and those are *thoughts*.

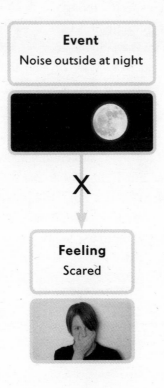

Identifying the thought: what made that noise outside?

Soon after a *situation* (in this example, a noise outside), and shortly before *feelings* (e.g. feeling 'scared'), there are *thoughts*. It can be really hard for adults, and therefore even harder for kids, to catch those thoughts that lead to feelings of being scared. So when discussing this with children, we need to be very specific. In this example, where the situation is a noise outside, it can lead to a specific question that attempts to catch specific thoughts. To support your child to identify their thoughts it is best to ask simple questions – 'What do you think made the noise outside to make you / George feel scared?' or, 'Why do you think you/George felt scared?' Usually, the first answer that comes to children's minds is 'Burglar' or 'Robber', but sometimes it can be 'Monster' or 'Alien'.

Once you have identified your child's 'worry thought', ask them to rate how much they think that thought is true. So if they think the noise is a burglar, how strongly do they think this from not at all (0) to definitely true (10). Below is a rating scale that you can use to help your child with this.

	Worry thoughts:	How true?
Example child	*There is a burglar outside who is going to break in and hurt me*	10/10
Your child		

How strongly does your child believe that this thought is true?

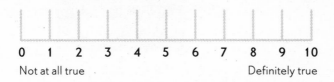

<table>
0   1   2   3   4   5   6   7   8   9   10
Not at all true   Definitely true
</table>

Believe it or not, it can be nice to respond with 'That makes sense.' We don't mean to reinforce kids' unpleasant thoughts, but what we do say is, 'If there is a noise outside, it makes sense that George would be scared *if* he thought it was a burglar that made the noise.'

In this activity, what you are trying to do is to reinforce the link between the situation (noise outside), the feeling (scared) and the thought (burglar). This way, your child begins to learn that feelings are not just random, but tied to both situations and thoughts.

The long-term goal is that when they have a strong feeling, and can think about what situation created that feeling, then they can try to remember what they were just thinking about. As you can see from the picture below, there is a final step. We ask children, 'If George is scared, does that mean he is going to feel awake or sleepy?' Now the child is connecting the situation, the thought and the feeling, and thinking about why it might mean it is harder to fall asleep.

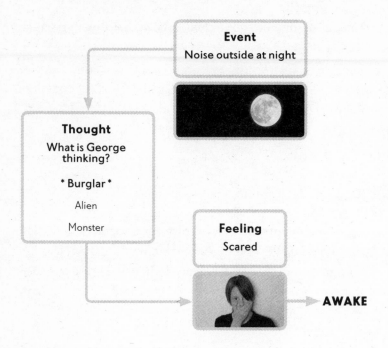

Changing worried/scared thoughts to more balanced thoughts

Once you and your child have identified their main 'worry thought(s)', the next step is then to practise challenging the thought that led to the feeling of being scared. The key to challenging a thought is not that it is 'bad' or 'wrong' but, rather, could there be another, more balanced way of thinking that might lead to a different feeling?

> *'Could there be another way of thinking that might lead to a different feeling?'*

In this case the thought is 'the noise outside is a burglar/ robber'. But what else might the noise be? Most children are able to answer this question, even with a little help. In the figure below is a list (in the Thought box) of common answers given by children.

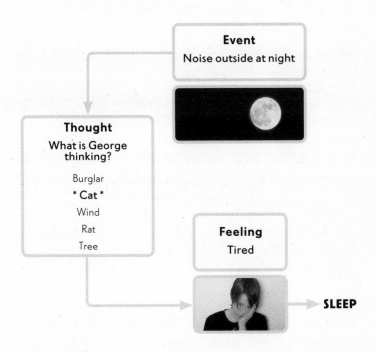

As soon as the child is able to give an alternative to 'burglar', stop for a moment, and say, 'So, before the noise was definitely made by a burglar. But now it might not be a burglar – it might actually be a cat.' This is the way we want children to begin to think. We want them to consider their initial thoughts in a more analytical way.

But don't stop there.

Keep asking your child: 'What else could have made the noise outside?' and 'Anything else?' or, 'When you have heard a noise outside your house before, what did you think it was?' Perhaps your child could go and ask other people in the family what they think – what does their other parent think could have made the noise? Or do their siblings or grandparents have any other ideas? The goal is to generate a list. A long list.

Looking over your list of all the possible different things that could have made the noise outside, direct your child to rate once more how true they think their original worry thought is. The goal is to show your child that there are lots of different ways to interpret the noise, so it cannot be 100 per cent true that it is a burglar.

Hopefully by now your child is understanding that the noise could have come from multiple sources. Now you might ask them what they think was *most* likely to have caused the noise.

More often than not, 'a cat' or 'the wind' rank the highest. Perhaps, even with an exhaustive list, they still think it is the burglar. If your child still identifies the burglar as the most likely option, ask them to also pick a second most likely option. Then the next step is to support your child to look for clues to decide what has made the noise.

> *'Support your child to look for clues to decide what has made the noise.'*

Why is it most likely to be a cat (or whatever they have identified)? How often do you hear noises outside? Has it ever been a burglar? Have you seen cats that live nearby?

Your child might discuss with you how cats can be nocturnal, how they know your neighbour has a cat that likes to visit your garden at night-time, or that the next morning the wind had blown some things around outside which shows the wind must have been responsible for making noises. In these cases, children are gathering facts to support their choices. Again, you might want to rope in some family members to help with this. Has their other parent ever heard noises outside at night-time? Has it ever been a burglar? Have they ever seen cats outside? What noises do leaves make in the wind? All of this information is to support your child to look at alternative explanations for their worry thought.

> *'Support your child to look at alternative explanations for their worry thought.'*

Finally, you will have a list of evidence for and against their worry thought and might also have a list of evidence to support their alternative explanations (e.g. that it was a cat). With all this information now in front of them, ask your child to identify what they think the most likely cause of the noise is. Hopefully, by this stage, they will be seeing that it is much more likely that it was a cat or the wind than it was a burglar.

Below is an example of a worksheet that you could use to help your child to look for clues about their worry thought (a copy can also be found in the Appendix, page 228). The goal is to generate a long list of clues that challenge their worry thought and might support a more balanced thought. You'll see on the worksheet that after generating the list of evidence for and against the worry thought, your child can then rate how true they think their original worry thought was. While we wouldn't expect it to go down to '0', the goal is that it has reduced, now that they are looking at the evidence against their worry thought and starting to think of more balanced thoughts.

Putting this all together

As a final step, run through the full sequence of events with your child's newly generated hypothesis (in this example – that the noise is a neighbourhood cat).

- Restate that a noise was made outside

- That George (or your child) thought it was a cat

- Ask your child how that would make George (or themselves) feel? (the answers are wide and varied, but not 'scared')

- We then ask, 'So if George is now feeling tired, is he likely to be Awake or Sleepy?'

Worry thought	How true?	Evidence for	Evidence against	How true now?	A balanced thought
There is a burglar outside who is going to get inside and hurt me.	9/10	My friend told me that her house was broken into. I've heard about burglars on the news.	Even though I've heard sounds outside lots of times, a burglar has never been in our house. Our neighbour has a cat that likes to play in our garden and could be making the sound. There are lots of animals that live outside and become more active at night-time – like hedgehogs and owls. Some nights it is windy and the wind might make noises in the trees near our house. Dad says that he has never seen a burglar at our house and the neighbours have never seen one either. There is no way for a burglar to get into our house because they can't get through the windows or doors.	3/10	The noise outside is probably the neighbour's cat running around.

No prizes for what the answer is.

Then again, sleep is a great reward!

Where To From Here?

Practise, Practise, Practise

Generating worry thoughts and looking for clues for and against particular thoughts can be challenging for children, and you will need to support them to practise this. As they practise more and more, the aim would be that they can quickly challenge these scary thoughts by themselves.

Developing more balanced thinking requires a lot of practice – in fact, many weeks of practice. We say to children that it's like learning your times tables. At first it seems like an impossible task, but after practising them over and over they can go through them, often without giving it much thought at all.

The 'Practise, Practise, Practise' idea is to:

1. Keep training your child to better catch and speak about their thoughts,

2. And then to come up with other thoughts (by using the 'What else?' type of questions and looking for clues about their thoughts).

So, these are great skills to practise during the day. Maybe over dinner, maybe in the car to school – practice will be what makes it develop as a skill that they can use at night-time (and even in other situations where they feel intense, unpleasant emotions). The more it is practised during the day, the more likely it will be that your child can access this new way of thinking at night-time. Sometimes the situation is not a noise outside, but instead your child sees a shadow 'creeping' across the bedroom. Again, you can use cognitive techniques to analyse your child's thoughts. Is it their eyes playing tricks on them? Like when we're travelling in a car at night and stare at the moon – believing it is following us home. Are there car lights moving outside that project dim light through curtains that make it seem like shadows are moving? Keep using questions to guide your child logically to the point where you can generate a list, so their initial thought of what might be scary is not 100 per cent true.

What If Your Child's Worry is Realistic?

For some young people, particularly older children, their worry can stem from very real friendship difficulties, school problems, family difficulties, or other concerns. In such cases, they may experience transient sleep difficulties that resolve when the problem resolves. However, it may act to precipitate a more chronic sleep problem. If the thoughts keeping your child awake at night are stemming from an actual problem, we would not recommend going down the path of looking for evidence for and against their thought. This is less likely to be a helpful strategy if their worry is indeed realistic. In these cases, it is better to support your child to problem-solve how they might manage such situations. For example, sit together and plan how your child (and you) could take actions to deal with the problem. You might generate a list of all of the possible ways you could deal with the problem and look at the pros and cons of each strategy. When you have decided on a strategy, you can then support your child to implement the strategy. Below is a possible template to use to support your child to think about what actions they or you might be able to take to help them with their problem. This is not an activity that should be done around bedtime as it could serve to exacerbate their night-time anxiety. However, this can be a very helpful activity to do together at another time, such as after school or at the weekend. Even if the worry seems small to you, doing some simple problem-solving can help your child to feel that their problem is valid and teach them ways to think about overcoming or solving the problem.

In cases of realistic worry, to target their sleep, Bedtime or Sleep Restriction techniques are still the recommended approach, as the increased sleep pressure will help them fall asleep quicker and to get a better-quality sleep. Many young people we have seen in our clinical work may be experiencing some friendship difficulties or worries about school – many might be described by their parent as a 'worrier' or 'over-thinker' in general. In these cases, we still follow the same sleep programme as has been described in this book, but might complete the problem-solving task instead of the worry thought task, if this additional section is necessary. However, if your child is experiencing high anxiety from realistic issues, such as friendship

What is the problem?			
		PROS	CONS
Action 1:			
Action 2:			
Action 3:			

problems, and this impacts on their well-being in general, you might find it useful to refer to books that go into detail about managing child anxiety more generally – we have provided Further Reading suggestions towards the end of this book.

5

Exposure: Helping Your Child to Face Their Fears Step By Step

In This Chapter:

- Understanding Exposure and rating emotions

- Developing Exposure ladders to support your child in facing their fears, step by step

- Developing rewards charts to motivate your child to face their fears

When to Use?

- Your child's sleep-related anxiety remains elevated

- If your child still wants you to be present for them to fall asleep or still wants to sleep in your bed/room

- Your child has completed either Bedtime or Sleep Restriction

What is Exposure?

In our clinical work, we find that many children are able to overcome their sleep problems after using either Bedtime Restriction or Sleep Restriction, without the need for any further intervention. Because they fall asleep more quickly, they learn that bed and sleep is a safe space. However, in some cases, there may be residual difficulties. For example, like with 6-year-old Sophie after Bedtime Restriction (Part II, chapter 3), your child may still be resistant to sleeping in their own bed, or falling asleep without a parent present. In such cases, your child may benefit from a technique called Exposure.

Exposure forms the basis of many evidence-based interventions for child (and adult) anxiety, and it is no different for anxiety around sleep.

Exposure is all about learning new skills. Like everything we learn, we get better with practice. Learning to go to school, learning to ride a bike, learning to like new foods. All of these are things you, and your child, have learned by being exposed to them, over and over again.

> 'Exposure is all about learning new skills. Like everything we learn, we get better with practice.'

Here, we have included an example that you can use to explain Exposure to your child. We use the example of a child who is scared of butterflies because most children know that butterflies aren't scary. If your child is a bit unsure of butterflies, you can change it to something else – something that they can obviously identify as *not* scary or a cause for anxiety. Here is the butterfly example that you can use to explain this to your child:

Chloe is scared of butterflies. She thinks that if a butterfly touches her skin it will bite her. Because she is worried about them she always stays far away from them. Sometimes she doesn't even want to go outside to play! But because Chloe never goes to see butterflies, she's never been able to learn that butterflies are safe. (If your child is old enough, you might want to ask them what they think the problem is with Chloe avoiding butterflies or what they might tell Chloe to do to overcome her fear – to help them generate the idea that avoiding something you're worried about means you cannot learn to 'un-worry'.) *Chloe really wants to overcome her worry about butterflies and so she and her dad set up a 'stepladder' of activities to help her face her fears.*

Step 1: *First, Chloe and her dad look at pictures of butterflies on the Internet. They learn lots of interesting facts about butterflies too [just like you have now learned lots about sleep].*

Step 2: *Chloe and her dad go out to the garden to look at butterflies together. Chloe watches butterflies land on her dad.*

Step 3: *Chloe and her dad go to a butterfly house so they can touch a butterfly. Chloe's dad stays with her. By now Chloe is learning that butterflies are safe.*

Step 4: *Chloe goes outside to look at the butterflies flying around, without her dad there. She has now learned that butterflies aren't dangerous and has overcome her fear!*

Like with learning that butterflies aren't dangerous, we can also help children to learn that sleeping on their own is safe. But first – some important steps.

Rating Emotions

As part of Exposure, children learn how to rate the strength of their feelings. To do this with your child you may want to use a 'feeling thermometer'. This involves helping your child to identify that a thermometer is used to measure how hot we are, from a normal temperature up to very, very hot (with gains in technology this is rarely what a thermometer looks like any more – but most children still understand this analogy). With a feeling thermometer you can teach your child to rate how strongly they are feeling a particular emotion. You will find an example of a feeling thermometer in the Appendix (see page 229).

Here are some practice questions to make sure they understand how to use it to rate how they feel.

1. How scared would you feel if you were on a giant rollercoaster?

2. How scared would you feel if there was a giant spider on your shoulder?

3.   How scared would you feel if you were watching
      your favourite movie?

Use the feeling thermometer to get your child to practise
rating their feelings, from 1 – *not at all* scared, to 10 – *very,
very* scared. This is to help them orientate to rating emotions differently depending on the situation.

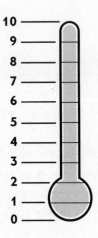

Beginning Exposure

Phase 1: Identifying a New Skill

Decide what skill you'd like your child to learn. Ideally,
you would do this in discussion with your child, although
ultimately you will need to decide what the end-goal is
(your child might be perfectly fine with sleeping in your

bed, and therefore not motivated to learn the new skill!). Some children (especially older children) will be very motivated to reach this goal – so they can go to sleepovers or school camps. Younger children may be initially resistant. Here's a common interaction we see:

Parent: *Wouldn't it be great if you fell asleep all by yourself in your bed like a big girl?*

Child: *No.*

While the bluntness of the above example is somewhat tongue-in-cheek, it is a common interaction that we see. Of course, you might be able to talk to your child about this in a way that shows them the advantages of reaching their goal. Perhaps they have wanted to be able to have a sleepover with their best friend, or be able to sleep in their own bed with their own special quilt/duvet cover. Either way, in these cases, you might have the ultimate goal in mind (i.e. the goal you set in Part II, chapter 2) but start with focusing on the smaller, or first steps, on your child's stepladder. Your child will feel more motivated if steps are achievable and linked to a reward. As their confidence and understanding of the reward system grows, you can move closer and closer to your ultimate goal.

With each step, use the feeling thermometer and get your child to rate how scared they currently are (0 = not at all scared, 10 = very, very scared).

Phase 2: Learning The New Skills

Over time we want to see this 'scared level' decrease, showing your child is less and less scared as they master their new skill.

How do they learn to be less scared? By breaking down their learning into smaller steps. You saw this in the butterfly example where Chloe started on a step where she only felt a little bit scared (looking at pictures of butterflies and then going outside, but with her dad present). To ensure each step is mastered, you should set an amount of times each step should be achieved and monitor how their anxiety reduces (e.g. step 1 is performed four times before moving to step 2, as their anxiety goes down from 6/10 to 3/10). The steps then get more and more challenging until your child reaches their ultimate goal. Later steps may take a few more tries to ensure their anxiety has come down to a manageable level.

If your child is particularly attached to one parent, it might be a useful tip to get the other parent to lead their new bedtime routine. For example, often in the clinic we see that the child is most upset when their mum will not stay with them. Therefore, we encourage the dad to be more involved in the stepladder – being the parent that sits in the room for the first few steps, for example. If this is possible/practical in your family, you might want to try it as an extra tip.

Choosing your steps

Work with your child to determine what each step will be, starting with something that is a little bit scary but manageable (maybe around a '3' on the feeling thermometer) and moving up to the ultimate goal (e.g. going to bed and falling asleep by themselves). Each step should be challenging for your child, as they are learning to face their fears. The specific steps will be different for each child. If your child needs you to be in their bed with them before they fall asleep, you might find that the first step on the ladder is to have you sitting at the end of their bed.

Clinically, we see better success if the stepladder can start in the child's own bed, even if the parent stays with them as the first step. In these cases, step 1 might be as straightforward as the child falling asleep with their parent sitting on a chair in the corner of the bedroom. Step 2 might be the child falling asleep with their parent sitting in the doorway, and Step 3 might be the child falling asleep with the parent standing in the hallway. However, if this is not possible, there is no reason the stepladder cannot start from the parents' bedroom. We have worked with children to move their mattress from their parents' bedroom to their own bedroom (something we jokingly coined 'mattress removal therapy'). If your child needs to be in your bed to fall asleep, the first step on the ladder may be them falling asleep on a mattress next to your bed. If they only feel settled to sleep if you pop your head around the door every few minutes, then the first step might be to pop your head around the door after 5 minutes, and gradually increase this timing.

Talk with your child to work out 4 or 5 steps that they can aim to achieve. The number of steps will depend on the level of their anxiety – the more anxious they are, the more steps they may need. Remember, at the beginning, it is likely that the final step should be rated as a '9' or '10' out of '10' on the feeling thermometer, as this is their (or your) ultimate goal. The general rule is that your child practises each step until their worry goes down to a '2' or '3' on the feeling thermometer, or until they can complete each step with minimal fuss or anxiety.

Like with the sleep diaries, it is important to record this information. You might use a ladder as an example of the child climbing steps towards their goal. Your child can then put this up on the fridge or in their room to allow them (and you) to monitor their progress. A copy of the ladder can be found in the Appendix (see page 230). Later in this chapter we'll take you through some sleep-related examples.

Phase 3: Supporting Your Child to Achieve the Goal

Your child is working towards overcoming their anxiety. An important way to support this is through encouragement and small rewards, as they achieve each step.

Key things about rewards:

1. The rewards are tied to *practising* steps

2. The rewards are more about 'doing things' and less

about 'having things' (e.g. going on a family outing, being able to choose a movie, picking their favourite meal for dinner). If there is a toy or game that is really motivating for them, you might keep it as a reward for the final step

3. The rewards must be something your child really wants and should get more exciting the harder the goals they achieve

4. The rewards should not be money

And, most importantly . . .

The rewards are always tied to praise and encouragement from the parent.

Setting up a visual reminder of their progress

When you and your child set up the steps of the exposure ladder, make sure to leave space to attach the reward to each step. When we go through examples below, you'll see a simple template of a stepladder with a rewards chart (and one can be found in the Appendix, page 230). But if you have time, it's a great idea to make this with your child so it can be more colourful and fun!

The reward should be tied to the level they are practising. For the first level, where they are completing a mild-anxiety task (e.g. the parent sitting in a chair next to the bed, or the child sleeping on a mattress on the floor in their

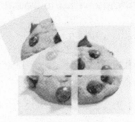

parent's/parents' bedroom), the reward for this step may be helping the parent make chocolate-chip cookies at the weekend (or some other treat the child loves). Your child needs to achieve and practise this step a certain number of times to receive this reward. A general guideline is to complete the step four times. One idea may be to print off a picture of a cookie and cut it into four pieces. Each time your child achieves the first step, they add a piece of the cookie. When the cookie is complete, it is time for their reward! Or perhaps they will receive a stamp on the page each time they achieve success, and after four stamps they receive their reward. This way they can monitor their progress. Some nights they might not achieve the step. In this example that means they don't get a stamp or a piece of the cookie added (but they don't lose a piece either). The message should be that, even if they stumble on the chart, they can always be encouraged to try again the next night.

The child will then move up their ladder, receiving their reward for each achievement. The reward for the final step should be the biggest one. Examples might be:

- having a friend to stay for a sleepover

- going to the cinema with the parent

- going on a family outing

- getting a toy or new game that they really want

Each reward needs to be motivating for the child (within reason – no red Ferraris!).

Example: Sophie – 6 Years Old

You will remember Sophie from the previous section, where she completed Bedtime Restriction, but still had some residual issues with anxiety around sleeping alone. Sophie would sleep in her own bed, but only if a parent was with her. Many nights she slept on a mattress in her parents' room. If she was put to sleep in her own bed, she used to wake during the night and go to her parents' room.

Via her Bedtime Restriction programme, Sophie now falls asleep by herself in her parents' room. She has even had some success falling asleep by herself in her own room, but overall is still very resistant to sleeping in her own bed. Sophie's sleep pattern is continued from her example in the previous section. She is falling asleep at 8.30 p.m. and wakes up at 6.30 a.m. and is therefore getting about 10 hours' sleep each night. This was judged as enough sleep for Sophie, who was functioning fine during the day. This same sleep schedule will continue, but she will also begin her steps on her Exposure ladder.

The ultimate goal for Sophie's Exposure ladder is to fall asleep in her own bed without her parents being present. Sophie's parents want her back in her own bed but Sophie will only do this if they are present. Before they begin to identify steps in the ladder, her mum goes back over the butterfly example so that Sophie understands the idea of facing her fears and building things up slowly. They then start to work out the steps. For the first step, Sophie wants to fall asleep in her own bed with her mum lying with her. This is a '0' on her feeling thermometer – she is not scared at all. Together they think of a first step about which she feels 'a little bit' scared. Her first step will be to fall asleep in her own bed with her mum or dad sitting on a chair next to the bed. It is very important that Sophie is clear what her first step is. Her mum or dad will be on a chair next to her bed, but they will not be talking. It is quiet time to fall asleep. If Sophie achieves the step, she gets a stamp on her rewards chart. They decide that once she gets four stamps she gets her reward.

The goal of her following steps is for her parent to move further and further away, until it is no longer necessary for a parent to be in her room when she falls asleep.

Sophie's Exposure Ladder

STEPS:

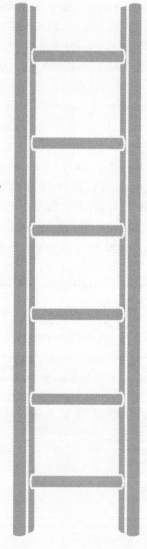

5. Go to sleep on own in own bed

4. Go to sleep with parent in next room/ standing in kitchen

3. Go to sleep with parent a few rooms away but they look in to her room every few minutes

2. Go to sleep with parent standing in doorway, facing away

1. Go to sleep in own bed with parent sitting on chair next to her bed

Sophie's Reward Ladder

STEPS:

REWARDS:

5. Go to sleep on own in own bed

5. Get to choose a toy from toyshop

4. Go to sleep with parent in next room/ standing in kitchen

4. Have cousin to sleep over

3. Go to sleep with parent a few rooms away but they look in to her room every few minutes

3. Go to the cinema with parent

2. Go to sleep with parent standing in doorway, facing away

2. Have a special movie night with Mum and Dad

1. Go to sleep in own bed with parent sitting on chair next to her bed

1. Bake favourite cake

Step 1 (nights 1–4):

Sophie moves through the first step easily, falling asleep with her parent sitting on a chair next to her bed. This is a good thing as it has allowed her to actually see the connection between reaching the step and getting her reward. Even though her parent is sitting there, they are not communicating. Over breakfast, they get out the feeling thermometer and Sophie rates how scared she feels as a '1' or '2', showing this step is an easy one for her to tackle. At the weekend she makes a chocolate cake with her dad.

Step 2 (nights 5–8):

For the next four nights, Sophie also achieves her goal, and falls asleep each night with her parent standing in the doorway, facing away from the room. On the first night, her worry is a '4' on the scale, but after doing this step for four nights, she rates it at a '2'. She picks out her favourite movie and gets to buy some popcorn for a family movie night at the weekend.

Step 3 (nights 9–12):

Step 3 is a bigger step for Sophie as she cannot see her parent. However, by now she has a good understanding of getting the reward for achieving the step and she is very motivated to receive this reward. The first night on this step, Sophie is nervous (rates a '7' on her thermometer). Sophie asks her mum to bring the chair back into her bedroom so

her mum can sit on it. Her mum reminds her about working towards going to the cinema (her Step 3 reward) and,
at this stage, that is enough for Sophie to go to sleep. On
the first night she calls out to her parents and they respond
by saying 'two minutes'. Then, after this time, they pop
their head around the door (giving a reassuring smile, but
making no conversation), then go back to the room next
door. After another few minutes they repeat this, but by
the third time, Sophie is asleep. Unbeknown to Sophie,
they extend the period before popping back in each time,
meaning that Sophie is in bed without her parent present
for longer. Sophie continues to seek some reassurance on
the second night, but by night three, as her sleep pressure
builds, Sophie stays in her bed and has stopped calling out.
Usually, by the second time Sophie's parent pops into her
room, she is asleep anyway, showing her anxiety is reducing. By the final night of this step, Sophie rates her worry
as a '2'.

Step 4 (nights 13–15/16):

The last two steps are more challenging again for Sophie,
as she can no longer see her parent. Her parent makes some
soft sounds now and then outside her room (although not
directly at Sophie), so she knows that for the most part
they are nearby. But the pauses between these soft sounds
gradually get longer and longer. Sophie initially rates her
worry as a '7' on the thermometer because she won't be
able to see her mum or dad. However, her mum and dad
remind her that before they even started the stepladder she

was already being a *Sleep Ninja*! She had already slept for many nights all by herself. For two nights, Sophie achieves her goal of falling asleep in her bed with her parents out of the room (but still standing in the next room or hallway so she can hear them now and then).

On the third night there is a small setback. Sophie does not want to fall asleep without her parent in her room. She gets out of bed to try to get her mum to sit in her room. Sophie's dad leads Sophie back to her bed each time, avoiding too much fuss. He puts her back in bed, says goodnight and leaves the room. This happens twice until Sophie falls asleep. This was a difficult night as Sophie became upset. But her dad stuck consistently to guiding her back to her own bed. The next day Sophie doesn't get a stamp on her chart – but she can try again the next night and they tell her that they are proud about how hard she is trying to face her worry. They even talk about it on the way to school, and her mum reminds her of how well she has been doing. The next two nights Sophie achieves her goal of four nights sleeping alone with her parents in the next room.

Sophie gets to invite her cousin for a sleepover!

Step 5 (nights 17–20):

Sophie is now practising her final step of falling asleep in her own bed on her own. Her parents do not need to be in the next room or waiting in the hallway. Sophie completes all four nights in a row, and as a result can go to the toyshop for her reward.

Sophie is now not only sleeping from 8.30 p.m. to 6.30 a.m. each night, but is also going to sleep without a parent present.

Common Questions and Issues:

My child keeps getting out of bed.

Please refer to the earlier Common Questions and Issues section in Part II, chapter 3 (pages 73–86) where we have discussed this. The same response should be provided that we discussed around the sleep time interventions – that is, be calm and quietly take them back to their own bed, without fuss or over-reassurance. This is often what parents tell us they find most challenging in the sleep programme, but with persistence and consistency it can be very effective. Often, persistency for just two nights, even if those nights are very difficult, is enough to see large reductions in their nighttime resistance/worries.

My child seems to find the steps too easy.

Like there was in Sophie's case, often after Bedtime or Sleep Restriction there will be some improvement in their ability to sleep in their own room. Therefore, some of the first steps might be quite easy. This isn't a bad thing – it provides a nice opportunity for your child to learn about the reward system and experience achievement. That said, you and your child might decide you want to skip a step. For example, you and your child might decide to skip step 3 and go straight to step 4. Your child can then get both of their rewards in the same weekend, which can be quite enticing! Just make sure your child is ready to skip a step – use the feeling thermometer to check their anxiety around the steps. We don't want to set them up to fail.

My child is very scared of the last steps.

In the clinic, we often see a big jump in anxiety around the last few steps. Inevitably in these final steps the parent at some point cannot be present in the room (if this is the goal). This is why we often have a middle step – where the parent is still in the hallway (not in the room but also not too far away). If your child's anxiety is still high after four attempts on the higher step, it's fine to stay on this step for a bit longer until their anxiety goes down. For example, stay on the step where the parent is in the hall for another few nights, and then move on to the final step. You may also need to add another step in between to make the steps more manageable. Ultimately, for your child to overcome their fears, they must face them, and it is okay that this is difficult for them. Fear and worry are valid emotions and we certainly do not want to send children the message that they should never feel uncomfortable emotions. As part of Exposure, at some point your child will face fears that are difficult for them, but with your consistency and persistence they can be supported to overcome them, even if it does not feel possible at first. In Part I we talked about key traps that parents can fall into when trying to support their child's worries. This includes over-reassurance and supporting your child to avoid things they are afraid of. Instead, as outlined in Part II, chapter 3, if your child continues to get out of bed to seek assurance, follow a consistent pattern – walking them back to bed, tucking them in and leaving the room. Again, persistence and consistency is key.

My child doesn't meet their goal each night.

This is OK! No one sleeps perfectly every night and there can be some bumps along the road as we learn any new skill. After a 'bad night', remind your child of the success they've had. You might even want to pull out their sleep diary and show them how far they've come. Even though they won't get a stamp on their rewards chart the next day, the attitude should always be that they can try again the next night.

6

Relaxation Techniques

When we first began assessing our sleep interventions, through our clinical work and research, it usually included a component where we taught children some relaxation exercises. The idea was that this would give them something to do when they were feeling anxious. However, our research and clinical experience generally showed that these techniques were not as effective as the treatments we have already outlined in this book. When a young child is lying in bed and hears a noise outside, they generally just want to go straight to their parent, rather than try to do a breathing exercise! So it takes their parent, and the strategies we've already described, to help them to face their sleep-related anxiety.

Nevertheless, relaxation techniques certainly don't do harm and we know some children and parents particularly like this type of exercise, so we will briefly mention them here. Like with supporting your child to identify and challenge their worry thoughts, practice makes perfect when it comes to relaxation techniques. If you would like to help your child to use relaxation exercises, it is important that they are practised regularly, including at times when they are not anxious. If they don't practise them, it is unlikely that they would start automatically using them when they feel anxious. You might practise them on the way to school, over the breakfast table, or before they start their bedtime routine. Worksheets on mindful breathing exercises are readily available via a quick Internet search, but below are some brief examples.

If you want to introduce relaxation techniques to your child, do this at the beginning of the programme, so they can practise their night-time relaxation exercises from the beginning as they tackle their new bedtime routine.

Controlled Breathing

This method of relaxation is used in many clinical treatments for anxiety. If you search under 'Controlled Breathing' on the Internet, you will find plenty of advice on techniques and a range of specific exercises to follow. As we discussed in Part I, when we become anxious, our hearts beat faster, our blood starts pumping faster, our breathing gets faster. Controlled breathing aims to manage this, and when used with your child should help bring their breathing back under control and manage the feeling of anxiety. The technique is relatively simple – the child should breathe in slowly, counting to 5, hold, breathe out slowly, counting to 5. Repeat. Alternatively your child can take a deep breath, holding it in for 5 counts, and then slowly release the breath. Either is fine. The key is to slow the breathing (including the out-breath).

Controlled Breathing

- Breathe in, counting to 5

- Hold

- Breathe out slowly, counting to 5

Progressive Muscle Relaxation

As the name suggests, progressive muscle relaxation involves training your child to progress through each of their muscles, tensing them, and relaxing (releasing) them. The aim is to teach your child to relax their muscles and help them identify when they might be tensing (e.g. when they become anxious). This technique can be used alongside the Controlled Breathing. So you can instruct your child to tense the muscle as he or she breathes in, and release as they breathe out.

An example of steps for your child include:

- **Toes** – curl your toes, count in your head to 5, release

- **Legs** – squeeze your thighs, count to 5, release

- **Hands** – curl your hands into fists, count to 5, release

- **Arms** – tense biceps, count to 5, release

- **Stomach** – tense stomach muscles, count to 5, release

- **Shoulders** – raise your shoulders up to your ears, count to 5, release

- **Face** – scrunch your face, count to 5, release

The aim is for your child to practise these steps regularly and then use their relaxation technique if they begin to feel worried as they're trying to fall asleep. It might not be a worry about a robber or monster, it might be that they have trouble 'turning off' their mind.

PART III

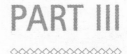

1

Helping Your Child with Parasomnias (e.g. Bed-Wetting, Night Terrors)

Sleep-walking, night terrors and bed-wetting (parasomnias) are other common sleep problems for children. Night terrors can be particularly distressing for the parent, as they involve the child abruptly 'waking' and screaming, appearing agitated and frightened. They may actually get out of bed and run around – as though they are extremely scared or 'stuck' in a nightmare. Despite all this distress, they are unresponsive to the parent's best efforts to comfort them. While this can be very upsetting for the parent, the child will commonly not remember anything about the incident when asked the next day. Sleep-walking can also be disturbing for the parent, who must be extra-vigilant that doors are properly locked and deadlocked, for fear the child might walk out of the house while they're asleep.

Although parasomnias most commonly occur during the toddler or pre-school years, sometimes they continue into early or later childhood. Sometimes your child may have insomnia (trouble falling asleep or waking during the night), and also the occasional parasomnia (e.g. night terror). In these cases, our research suggests that targeting the insomnia (using Bedtime Restriction, in Part II) is the best intervention. Bedtime Restriction should not dramatically restrict your child's sleep, but should improve the quality of the sleep. However, if parasomnias are your main concern (i.e. they occur most nights), then we would recommend trying the techniques outlined in this chapter.

Some parents we have seen have been told that their child will eventually grow out of their parasomnias (around the age of 10 years or so). For the most part, this is true. When children develop into young teenagers, there is a change in the intensity of their deep sleep. This developmental change typically takes place over a couple of years before this. So, your child will naturally develop less intense deep sleep, which coincides with a decrease in their parasomnias or bed-wetting. But, understandably, some parents do not wish to wait years until this developmental change occurs. It can be very disruptive and distressing to other family members when a child is having a night terror, and if bed-wetting persists, there can be significant stress and anxiety for children and parents – not to mention linen-washing.

Parasomnias generally occur during slow wave (deeper) sleep, and can be a consequence of sleep deprivation in children. Such sleep deprivation creates a more intense deep sleep; during this deep sleep, the body has a burst of activity that competes with that deep sleep and 'wakes' the child up. Parasomnias are actually relatively common in childhood, affecting up to 40 per cent of children at some stage. Because parasomnias occur in the deeper sleep stages, they tend to happen in the first third of the night (as we discussed in Part I). As children transition between different sleep stages, your child might get 'caught' between being asleep and awake, and present with behaviours that match both sleep (e.g. not responding, being difficult to wake) and wakefulness (e.g. walking or talking).

In this section, we will explain two interventions that may help your child – Scheduled Awakenings and Sleep Extension. Both have been shown to lead to reductions in (or even elimination of) parasomnias.

Scheduled Awakenings

When Should I Use Scheduled Awakenings?

Scheduled Awakenings should be used where parasomnias are the primary concern. This includes night terrors, sleep-walking or bed-wetting.

If you think your child is getting enough sleep but still has parasomnias, Scheduled Awakenings would be preferable to Sleep Extension. This is because your child is unlikely to get more sleep if they are already getting enough, making Sleep Extension futile. If you think your child seems very sleep deprived, please also read about Sleep Extension.

Why Should I Use It and How Does It Work?

Scheduled Awakenings work with your child's natural sleep cycles (as we discussed in Part I, chapter 1). The idea is to pre-empt the onset of your child's sleep issue (wetting the bed, night terror, walking in their sleep) by interrupting it and stopping it from happening. Fortunately it is a technique that you only need apply for 1–2 weeks.

Begin by using the sleep diary to establish your child's current typical sleep schedule (especially note how long it is after they fall asleep that the problem occurs – e.g. a night-terror). On the sleep diary, place a mark (e.g. 'N' for night terror; 'S' for sleep-walking) to show what time the parasomnia occurs.

Scheduled Awakening, Basic Steps

1. Work out the approximate time that your child's sleep problem occurs (usually within the first third of the night)

2. Pre-empt this by waking them 15–20 minutes before this time

3. Wake them gently, so they stir but are still sleepy

When you wake up your child, they should still be sleepy or 'groggy', as they have been woken up from their deep sleep. You might even find that they don't actually remember being woken up if you mention it the next morning. They shouldn't be completely woken up, to the point where they become very alert. They just need to be woken slightly – they may mumble something or seem confused.

The same principle applies for bed-wetting, but you will be taking them to the toilet during this wake-up. This can be tricky when they are very sleepy – they will probably need some careful directing! Ensure you plan this with your child so that they know the wake-up will be happening (the aim is not to frighten them!).

Scheduled Awakening

- No or minimal noise/talking

- Keep lights dim

- Aim for them to be slightly awake (still groggy and a bit floppy)

For night terrors or sleep-walking

- Sit them up in bed for a few minutes; you might just quietly say hello

- They should wake up (they might make a noise or mumble something) but should remain sleepy

- The aim is *not* to wake them up completely

Bed-wetting

- Limit any liquid intake in the hour or so before bed

- All of the above apply, but you should also help your child to go to the toilet. You will probably need to direct them there, as they will still be very sleepy.

Example: Harry – 8 Years Old, Night Terrors

Harry is 8 years old and experiences night terrors most nights. He usually falls asleep OK but often wakes up during the night, screaming as if he is being attacked. His parents have completed a sleep diary and established that Harry's night terrors occur about 2 hours after he falls asleep. He goes to sleep at 7.30 p.m. each night, so his night terror usually occurs around 9.30 p.m.

In some cases, a relatively quick and simple programme is enough to eliminate the parasomnia. Quite simply – Harry will be woken up 15–20 minutes before his average night-terror time, which will be around 9.10 to 9.15 p.m. This will continue for four days. If they are having success (i.e. his night terrors are reducing), then his parents will change the routine so they wake Harry up at around 9.15 p.m. every second night for the next four days. Next it will change to every third night, and so on, until Harry is sleeping through the night without any night terrors.

What About Bed-Wetting?

The same principle of Scheduled Awakening would apply for bed-wetting – wake your child 15–20 minutes before the bed-wetting is due, continue this for three of four days, then extend the programme so you wake them only every second night, then every third, then fifth, until they are sleeping through the night without experiencing any bed-wetting. For bed-wetting, when you gently wake them you can guide them (they should be sleepy) to the toilet to allow them to relieve themselves.

Sleep Extension

When Should I Use Sleep Extension?

- When parasomnias are the primary problem (e.g. sleep-walking, night terrors)

- Your child seems not to be getting enough sleep and is having problems with daytime functioning, such as feeling sleepy in class

Why Should I Use It?

Because sleep deprivation can be a cause of parasomnias, Sleep Extension is used to reverse these effects.

What Does It Involve?

As the name suggests, Sleep Extension is the reverse of Sleep

Restriction, with the main goal being to get your child to sleep longer. Sleep Extension is still a step-by-step process. You don't want to put your child to bed too early, as they'll probably just lie there awake. We certainly don't want to *cause* insomnia. So, as with Sleep or Bedtime Restriction, we usually move bedtimes in 15-minute intervals.

For example, if your child is sleeping from 9 p.m. to 7 a.m. and experiences night terrors, start putting your child to bed at 8.45 p.m. Continue with this bedtime for a week. If you do not see any difference in the frequency of their parasomnia, then move their bedtime by a further 15 minutes earlier, so that bedtime becomes 8.30 p.m.

As their sleep extends, you should notice that their parasomnia reduces in frequency, until it is no longer present.

When Do You Stop?

The optimal time is when your child gets to a bedtime when they fall asleep easily (e.g. under 20 minutes) and parasomnias are no longer present.

Other Options For Bed-Wetting

- Bed alarms – Research studies have shown that bed alarms can be effective in treating bed-wetting. When the bed alarm detects moisture, it sounds an alarm to wake the child up. The effectiveness of bed alarms is based upon learning theory. That is, over time, the child's brain associates the sensation of needing to go to the toilet with waking up from sleep. Although bed alarms help a lot of children (65–80 per cent of children), they will not be effective for every child.

- Daytime bladder exercises – a couple of exercises performed during the day may assist to strengthen your child's overall bladder control. First, when your child goes to urinate, they can try stopping mid-stream for a few seconds, and then recommence. Second, they can gradually delay the time they go to the toilet – initially from 15 to 30 seconds building up to a few minutes. You may find that these techniques help to reduce the number of accidents, but also remember that at night-time they will not have conscious control over their bed-wetting.

If you find that the Sleep Extension or Scheduled Awakenings techniques have not resolved your child's parasomnia, then it is recommended that you visit your family doctor and ask for a referral to a specialist sleep service, which can organise an overnight sleep study, where the child's brainwaves and other behaviours may be observed.

Responding to the Parasomnia

Even with significant improvement, sometimes the parasomnia can still occur every once in a while. In these instances we would recommend that you:

- Make sure your child is safe (e.g. lock outside doors;

install a child-proof gate near stairs if the parasomnia is sleep-walking).

•   Do not try to suddenly wake them. Remember, even if it doesn't look like it, they are asleep. Waking them is likely to cause them distress.

•   Provide a calm environment for them to 'ride out' their parasomnia until they fall back asleep.

•   Do not add to your child's feeling of shame or embarrassment. It goes without saying that many children feel a lot of shame over bed-wetting. However, bed-wetting is a parasomnia and is really out of their control. It is important that they understand this. You may remind them that lots of children experience bed-wetting at some point – probably other children in their class, but they just don't know about it.

Maintaining Good Sleep Practices

Congratulations! You have now learned a number of really important and effective techniques to help your child sleep better. So let's summarise the main points of what we hope you have learned:

1. Many school-aged children sleep poorly, and require their parents to be nearby to help them fall and/or return to sleep.

2. Anxiety can work in opposition to sleep, including when children are awake in bed at night and begin to worry. Building up sleep pressure can be a good 'opponent' to tackle anxiety.

3. Allowing your child to avoid their fear (e.g. letting them sleep in your bed each night) and over-reassuring them can serve to maintain their anxiety in the longer-term.

4. Monitoring your child's sleep with a sleep diary can be an effective way to monitor the effectiveness of the healthy sleep changes you make.

5. Bedtime Restriction or Sleep Restriction can be quick and powerful behavioural techniques to help your child fall asleep and stay asleep.

6. If your child still experiences anxiety at night, or they still need you nearby so they can sleep, you should try challenging worry thoughts (Part II, chapter 4, especially for children 8+ years old) and facing their fears step by step (Part II, chapter 5, for children of any age).

7. Scheduled Awakenings or Sleep Extension can be used to reduce your child's parasomnias.

Once you have supported your child to overcome their sleep problem, there is every chance that their good sleep will be maintained and there will be no further issues. However, sometimes busy lives mean sleep routines can be forgotten, bedtimes and wake-up times can be stretched, and you might notice some problems starting to reappear. They may become more resistant to going to sleep, wake in the night more than usual or look more tired in the morning.

This is no reason to panic – the skills you have learned in this book means you have the tools to get your child's sleep back on track. As your child gets older, their sleep needs will also change; if you notice some old problems re-emerging, simply use the sleep diary techniques to have a look at how bedtime/wake-up times might need to be shifted to support your child to have good-quality sleep.

To help maintain good sleep, we particularly recommend that you:

1. Make sure your child has a sleep routine that can be stuck to as consistently as possible.

2. For older children: keep practising thought challenging with your child to support them to come up with more balanced thoughts and to allow this to become part of their way of thinking.

3. Help your child to face their fears. Make sure you are not (even unintentionally) giving them the opportunity to avoid situations that they are unsure about.

The Boomerang Sleep Problem

Sometimes, sleep problems can return.

Sometimes they may be fairly easy to spot, because they have been preceded by a stressful event (death of a family member), or some other trigger (e.g. mild sickness), that has led to your child's sleep worsening.

Other times, sleep problems creep up slowly on children and their parents. This could be because when a child's sleep is no longer monitored regularly, bedtimes can become more erratic; children might also not have used their cognitive or exposure skills in a while and have reverted to some old habits.

In any case, it's important to fill out a new sleep diary, as this can provide some useful information. See if you can compare this to an old sleep diary that showed your child was sleeping well. It may even show a different bedtime to what they have now, or some irregularity to their bedtimes.

Because you've already practised some of these techniques in this book, it's likely that you'll turn to the ones that were successful for your child. Ask yourself some quick questions:

- Was Bedtime or Sleep Restriction helpful? If so, try one of these again.

- Did my child's sleep problem get better after they practised their cognitive and/or exposure skills? Again, try these if needed.

We should note that every single child eventually goes through some relatively large changes in their sleep. And these changes can be notoriously hard to spot because they gradually change over months and years as your child becomes a teenager.

3

A Note on Sleep in Adolescence

There are a number of experiences across the human lifespan that can change good sleep to bad. In adulthood, this can be around the birth of a child (where many parents report waking up more, not getting enough sleep, and their sleep becoming 'lighter'), menopause (more frequent waking during the night), and even retirement (a relaxing of a routine can gradually convert solid sleep to broken sleep).

One of those sleep-impacting life experiences is just around the corner for your child: adolescence. The beginning of adolescence is a particular challenge for two reasons. Most influentially, the onset of puberty changes the underlying biological sleep processes of your child. The second, closely related reason is that your child moves from primary school to secondary school. We thought we would dedicate the final chapter to this transitional event, so parents can be forewarned and ready, if and when a child's settled sleep patterns worsen when entering the teenage years.

As we have mentioned previously, when our sleep clinic opened over a decade ago, we noticed that children from pre-school age to pre-adolescence had a tendency to depend on their parents' presence in order to fall asleep (and stay asleep).

But we also noticed a sleep pattern among the teenagers who began to attend our clinic: they were commonly taking a long time to fall asleep. In contrast to school-aged children, once the teenagers were asleep, they generally stayed asleep. However, they took a *really* long time to fall asleep. In fact, most of them were falling asleep after their parents did, and finding it almost impossible to wake up in the morning. And the older these teenagers were, the later they were falling asleep. Many teenagers were falling asleep past midnight on school nights, and nearly 1 in 5 of them had a sleep problem so bad that it was leading to problems with school attendance.

> *'Many teenagers were falling asleep past midnight on school nights...'*

So the aim of this chapter is to teach you to recognise some early signs of this new type of sleep problem, known as Delayed Sleep-Wake Phase Disorder, just in case it is one that your child develops, and also to provide some tips to help prevent it.

Sleeping Too Little and Too Late

Adolescent sleep expert Professor Mary Carskadon perfectly summed up teenagers' sleep in a talk she gave in Adelaide, Australia. She titled the talk, '*Teen Sleep: Too*

Little and Too Late'. Perhaps it should have been the other way round – that is: too late and too little. Because when children become teenagers, they typically begin to fall asleep later. And when they fall asleep later on school nights, this leaves them not enough time to get good-quality sleep before the alarm goes off on school mornings. Thus, they fall asleep *too late*, and get *too little* sleep.

In our book, we have outlined two simple behavioural strategies – Bedtime Restriction and Sleep Restriction. Both of these techniques share the common tip of delaying children's bedtime to a later time, so that they build up enough sleep pressure, feel sleepier, and fall asleep quicker. These techniques rely on children's ability to build up sleep pressure, but when children become teenagers, their ability to build up sleep pressure begins to reduce.

> *'When children become teenagers, their ability to build up sleep pressure begins to reduce.'*

For example, as a 10 year old, Thomas was able to build up sleep pressure so that the later he went to bed, the more easily he was able to fall asleep. But this was before Thomas began to go through puberty. As he progresses through puberty, his later bedtime will no longer work for Thomas. So, by the age of 16 years, he will begin to take a long time to fall asleep again. This could be 30 minutes, 45 minutes, or even longer. Unless Thomas tells his parents he has trouble falling asleep, they will not know, as they will normally be asleep before he is. Therefore, Thomas's parents might see changes in his behaviours *on school mornings*, including him:

- Snoozing his alarm

- Sleeping through his alarm

- Needing his parents to help him wake up and get him out of bed

- Just not being himself – that is, not saying much, not having much expression on his face, being more irritable than usual

- *And at weekends*, sleeping in . . . a lot!

Of course, many of these behaviours are very common in teenagers. We would consider this to be a problem if lots of these behaviours appeared most mornings and didn't seem to be improving (for example, does not resolve itself after a stressful event – perhaps submitting a big assignment – has passed) and if the teenager is very difficult (sometimes impossible) to wake in the morning, meaning that they are often late for school.

In the example of Thomas, his inability to fall asleep at an appropriate time is not necessarily his fault. Although many people blame teenagers' technology use for their bad sleeping habits, a more likely reason for their sleep problem will be biological issues, not their behaviours. For teenagers, difficulty sleeping can also be due to increased stress associated with school workload or worries about friendships (Hiller et al., 2014).

Sleep Pressure Reduces as You Become a Teenager

In the 1970s, Professor Mary Carskadon ran what is now known as the Stanford Summer Sleep Camps (Carskadon et al., 1980). Young teenagers, who had not yet reached puberty, were invited to take part in a summer camp, where by day they performed a lot of fun activities, and then by night their sleep was monitored using sophisticated sensors and video cameras. And because it was during the summer break so there was no school, they were allowed to sleep for a maximum of 10 hours! Each summer thereafter, these teenagers were invited back to the Stanford Summer Sleep Camp. And each summer, their sleep was measured, year after year. There were quite a number of interesting findings from this study, but we are going to focus on two of them.

First, as these teenagers grew older, their sleep did not become 'too little'. In fact, it was quite stable. For each and every year that they were given a 10-hour opportunity to sleep, these teenagers managed to get 9.25 hours of sleep. This goes against what we usually see when we survey teenagers across adolescence, and indeed, across the world. What usually happens is that teenagers seem to get less and less sleep the older they get, and in some regions (e.g. North America, Asia), teenagers get even less sleep (Gradisar et al., 2011b). But they get less sleep on school nights. That is the key difference.

Second, these teenagers who attended the Stanford Summer Sleep Camps got 40 per cent less deep sleep as they grew older. You may recall that we have mentioned that sleep pressure is related to deep sleep. Well, it appears that with less deep sleep there is also a reduction in being able to build up sleep pressure. This was best observed by a 2005 study by Professor Mary Carskadon's research group (Taylor et al., 2005) which showed that older teenagers took a lot longer to fall asleep than younger teenagers – but this only occurred around the times of 10.30 p.m. to 2.30 a.m. (and assuming that they woke up that morning at 8 a.m.). Before 10.30 p.m., both younger and older teenagers were similarly alert, and after 2.30 a.m., both younger and older teenagers were similarly sleepy. So between 10.30 p.m. and 2.30 a.m. seems to be a time zone when older teenagers start to become more alert than they used to when they were younger. This means that as your child becomes a teenager, they may feel less sleepy from 10.30 p.m., and therefore might either take longer to fall asleep, or eventually learn that they may as well stay up later until they feel sleepy.

There is no 'cure' for a reduction in sleep pressure. But we do have a couple of good solutions for another biological reason for teenagers' poor sleep.

Catching Up: The Weekend Sleep-In

Another important biological reason for teenagers sleeping too little and too late is the timing of their internal body clock. For the vast majority of school-aged children, their body clock dictates that they fall asleep and wake up at times that align with what they need to do. That is, most children will not need an alarm clock to wake them up in the morning to go to school. However, teenagers gradually become more dependent on being woken by their alarm clock as they get older. This can be due to the timing of their body clock becoming later and later.

So how does a teenager's body clock become later?

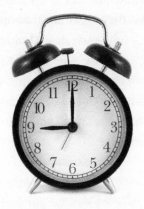

The Swiss pride themselves on creating clocks that take a perfect 24 hours to cycle through one day. For some reason, our own body clocks do not necessarily go through a perfect 24-hour cycle. Again, as with our height, weight and sleep need, we all differ in how long it takes for our body clock to complete one full cycle. Some people take less than 24 hours to complete a cycle, and they are usually older people. These older adults tend to struggle to stay awake in the evening, and wake up very early. In fact, over the years, we have even seen the same type of 'early sleeping pattern' (also known as 'morning larks') in several school-aged children in our Child & Adolescent Sleep Clinic. But other people, usually younger adults, have a body clock that goes for slightly longer than 24 hours. A Harvard University study showed that, on average, people had a body clock that cycled for 24.18 hours (or 24 hours and 11 minutes) (Czeisler et al., 1999). This means, if they do not implement a consistent daily routine, and instead go to sleep when they feel like it, and wake up when they feel like it, their bedtime and wake-up time will get later – delay – by 11 minutes each day. This equates to delayed sleep times of 77 minutes over 1 week, 308 minutes (or 5 hours and 8 minutes) over a month, and would even see their sleep patterns delay so much that they would eventually 'go around the clock' and return to their normal bedtime after 4.7 months.

'As with our height, weight and sleep need, we all differ in how long it takes for our body clock to complete one full cycle.'

So one theory is that the time it takes for a teenager's body clock to go through a full cycle is longer than 24 hours. This then creates a battle between the teenager's biology and the need to get up at the same time for at least five out of seven mornings a week to attend school.

Another possibility is that teenagers' body clocks are not considerably longer than 24 hours but, because of various influences, the timing has simply shifted later. One of the major influences is that body-clock timing can be shifted by bright light. Without going into too much technical detail, bright light *late in the evening* can delay the timing of the body clock. When humans are looking at bright light in the evening, it sends messages through the eyes and to the brain that they should be awake. Conversely, the absence of bright light *in the morning* – that is, being in dim light, darkness and even being asleep (when the eyes are not receiving any light) – can also delay the timing of sleep. In this way, it can delay the time a teenager wakes up, as well as delay the time they fall asleep at night. It delays their whole 24-hour rhythm.

Immediately, some parents will think that teenagers should avoid screenlight late at night, such as that from the screens of TVs, computers and phones. However, as we've previously discussed, the scientific findings have been mixed about whether it has a deleterious effect. But, considering teenagers' biology is already making them feel more alert, and newer technologies offer options for removing 'blue light' from screens, avoiding bright light (e.g. from laptop screens) is generally still recommended as good sleep hygiene.

Along with reducing bright light in the evenings, the absence of light in the morning means that teenagers' body clocks can delay in their timing. Certainly, when teenagers are asleep they are not getting light. This includes when they are sleeping in at weekends. Research has shown that when teenagers sleep in during a single weekend, they can delay the timing of their body clocks by an average of

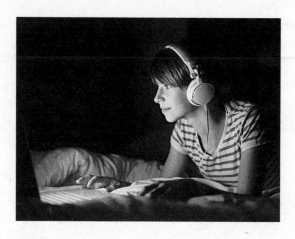

45 minutes (Crowley & Carskadon, 2010). Therefore, sleeping in can make teenagers' body-clock timing worse.

Of course, this is a catch-22. Having a big weekend sleep-in likely further assists with delaying your teen's body clock. If we think of the fuel-station example of sleep pressure from Part II, chapter 3, the later your teen sleeps in at the weekend, the longer they will need to be awake that day to build their sleep pressure, and the later they will fall asleep the next night. And so the delay continues or worsens. Yet, on the other hand, teenagers who sleep in at weekends probably do this because they are getting too little sleep on school nights, and therefore need to 'catch up' on their sleep. If they don't, then they may suffer significant consequences from continually getting too little sleep (Baum et al., 2014; Dewald et al., 2012; Lo et al., 2016; Short & Louca, 2015). So there is a fine line between allowing such teenagers to catch up on their sleep, yet not allowing them to sleep in too much. We discuss this in more detail below, with our tips for managing adolescent sleep.

Chicken or the Egg? Sleep Pressure or the Body Clock? We do not yet know which biological process changes first when children become teenagers. It could be that the body clock begins to delay later and later, and then children's sleep pressure begins to reduce. Or it could be that children's sleep pressure first reduces, meaning teenagers are staying up later, and then they are sleeping in as much as possible to try to catch up. And, in doing so, their body clocks are becoming later. Right now, we do not have well-developed scientific information to answer this question. However, our own research and the research of others continue to explore this question, so hopefully in a few years we will have an answer to how biology is affecting teenagers' sleep as they develop.

Is a Child Who Has Suffered Sleep Problems Going to Become a Late-Sleeping Teen?

After we treated about 42 school-aged children in our first trial of therapy for sleep problems, we followed up their progress a few years later. Unfortunately, we were unable to contact a lot of them for various reasons, but we managed to find and collect sleep data from 15 of them when they were 12 to 19 years of age. While a couple of the children now qualified as the type of late-sleeping teen that we have written about in this chapter, pleasingly, most of the children who had completed treatment using the techniques described in this book had been able to maintain their good sleep practices. This makes sense, as the reasons behind the sleep problems of the anxious child and those of the late-sleeping teen are quite different. The former usually have a body clock that is timed correctly, yet the latter have a body-clock timing that means their body wants to naturally wake up mid-morning when the school day is well under way. This means the techniques we have described in this book will not work for the late-sleeping teen. But don't lose hope; there are some solutions now and hopefully in the future.

Parent-Set Bedtimes

From 2008 to 2010, our research group conducted a large study of adolescents' sleep in Australia. The original purpose was to get a picture of what current sleep patterns were like in Australian adolescents. One of our researchers, Dr Michelle Short, had three teenagers of her own at the time. One night she asked one of her teenage sons to go to bed at a certain time, and he asked why; she told him she was pretty sure there was evidence to show that a specific bedtime aided better sleep and more efficient functioning the next day. When her son asked for chapter and verse on the research, she realised there was actually no published scientific evidence. So Dr Short tried to find an answer herself.

Sure enough, she was able to find that those teenagers who had an agreed bedtime with their parents not only slept more, but also experienced less fatigue the next day (Short et al., 2011). Around the same time, other researchers in the USA were finding parent-set bedtimes were also beneficial for teenagers' mood (Gangwisch et al., 2010). On average, only 18 per cent of Australian teenagers had bedtimes set by their parents, and this was generally on school nights. Yet it was much higher for teens in the USA (National Sleep Foundation; see Figure 4). Finally, and unsurprisingly, teenagers who had bedtimes set by their parents were generally younger than those who did not.

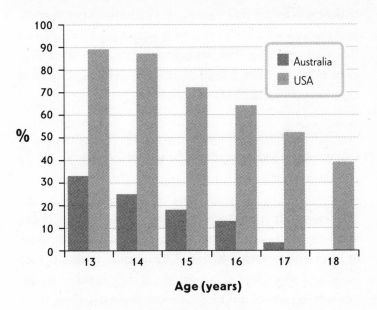

Figure 4 *Percentage of Australian and USA teenagers who had a parent-set bedtime.*

Fortunately if you are reading this book now, it is likely that the son or daughter whose sleep problems are concerning you is not yet a teenager. And the chances are that you have a set bedtime for your child (at least on school nights). So you have the opportunity to prevent, or at least minimise, sleep problems in your child as they become a teenager – we strongly urge you to set a consistent bedtime for them on school nights for as long as possible. As they progress through their school years, expect that they will naturally become more alert (because their biological sleep pressure is changing), so make the bedtime later, but still make them aware that they have a bedtime. At weekends, you can still set a bedtime, and it would be sensible to set this a bit later than their school-night bedtime. The difference between their school-night and weekend bedtimes should be within 2 hours of each other.

> *'The difference between their school-night and weekend bedtimes should be within 2 hours of each other.'*

Likewise, your young teenager may begin to sleep in longer and later at weekends. Ensure that they are still woken up at weekends within 2 hours of their usual wake-up time on school mornings. For example, if they usually get up at 7 a.m. on school mornings, ensure you wake them up at weekends before 9 a.m.

These strategies should work for most teenagers – and, in this case, prevention is better than a cure. That is, if you already have teenage children who do not have a set bedtime, you are likely to have considerable difficulty suddenly setting them a new bedtime on school nights. Nevertheless, it is worth having a conversation with them about the benefits of getting enough sleep (better school functioning, feeling happier, for example). Then you can negotiate a bedtime to help protect their sleep. You may even want to propose trialling it for a couple of weeks to see if they notice any benefits.

If you know ahead of time that you will not be able to have such a 'parent-set bedtime' conversation with your teen, then we would advise that you follow our earlier advice about waking them at weekends no later than 2 hours past their usual wake-up time on school mornings.

These measures are meant to prevent, or at least minimise, the severity of a teen sleep problem that can result from a delayed body clock. But it is just one technique among many. The next topic is one that we get asked about by many parents, teachers, health professionals and the media. What about the effect of technology on teenagers' sleep? The answer may surprise some people.

The Use of Technology

Many people may suggest that one of the best tips to help their teenage children sleep better is to remove all technological devices from their bedrooms. However, our research shows that technology use, in general, does not play a big role in harming young people's sleep. You might find that hard to believe, but we have done *a lot* of research into technology use and teenagers' sleep over the past several years. We admit that there will be some teenagers whose sleep is severely affected by technology use – but they are in the minority. Very interactive technologies (including social media) should also be avoided in the lead-up to bed. However, in general, technology use has less than 2 per cent influence on adolescents' sleep. Watching TV has virtually no influence on young people's sleep. There are other factors that influence the sleep of teens more, and many of these are within the family's control. As mentioned above, we recommend focusing on setting a bedtime for teenagers on school nights for as long as possible. This will play a bigger role in protecting your child's sleep as they become teenagers. Families can also provide a good sleeping environment, where the household is calm, quiet and easy-going. A lot of chaos, commotion and stress within a family can all impact negatively on a teenager's sleep. A hectic family lifestyle and lack of parent-set bedtimes actually contributes more to a teenager's sleep problem than the use of technology. So take a step back, have a look at how your household behaves in the evening, and see if you need to make any positive changes to your home in order to help your teen sleep better.

Natural Solutions to Help Teenagers Sleep Longer

It would take another whole book to explain sleep strategies for teenagers in detail, and would take more of an understanding of some of the factors causing poor sleep, aside from the biological ones explained above. The biological processes would also need to be described more fully, so that the treatments would make more sense. To give one example, however: although restricting your son or daughter's weekend sleep-in is helpful in preventing a serious delay of their body clock (and thus causing a serious sleep problem), it is also very important that teenagers get bright light in the morning.

This might sound strange – why would getting bright light in the morning help a teenager fall asleep quicker at night?

Just as our ears have two purposes (i.e. hearing and balance), our eyes also have two purposes. One obvious purpose is to see things or, more specifically, to allow our brain to receive visual information about the world around us. The optic nerves at the back of each of our eyes send this visual information to the back of our brains to process and make sense of what we are seeing. However, these optic nerves happen to pass really close to the home of the body clock, in the centre of our brains, in an area known as the supra-chiasmatic nucleus (or SCN for short). But it is not the visual information that the body clock is interested in, but more whether our eyes are seeing light or darkness.

If the body clock sees light, it suggests that it is daytime and that we should be awake. Conversely, if the body clock sees darkness, it suggests it is night-time and that we should be asleep.

This should make sense, especially given most of us feel sleepy when it is night-time, and become alert in the morning when the sun is rising.

So now, imagine your teenager has a sleep problem, where they are naturally falling asleep quite late (1 a.m.) and, if allowed to sleep in, would wake up late (e.g. 10 a.m.). When they sleep in until 10 a.m. on a Sunday morning, their eyes are closed, therefore their body clock sees darkness and informs the body that it should be asleep. When the teenager opens their eyes and the body clock begins receiving light, the body clock sees that the day has begun. This is when the body clock starts its timing (like pressing the start button on a stopwatch) and the teenager starts their day. Thus, the second purpose of our eyes is to help us reset our body clock.

The body clock does not know, or care, about what the actual time is. What is more important to the body clock is whether it is day or night. Thus, if it begins timing at 10 a.m. on a Sunday morning, the body clock expects that the teenager should fall asleep around 1 a.m. However, because it is Sunday night and school is starting at 8.30 a.m. the next day, parents, and even the teenager themselves, know they need to fall asleep early enough (e.g. 10–11 p.m.) in order to get enough sleep. So what happens? The teenager goes to bed at a 'decent' time (e.g. 10.30 p.m.), turns off all electronics, switches off the light, and . . . remains wide awake, for hours. They eventually fall asleep at 1 a.m. when their body clock is ready.

The good news is that there has been a lot of research over the last 30 years that can help us understand what happens to teenagers' sleep, and – particularly over the past 10 or so – we have begun to develop effective ways to treat the more severe sleep problems that affect teenagers. One of these methods is to trick the body clock about when it receives light and when it receives darkness, so that eventually the teenager falls asleep earlier and wakes up earlier. So ensuring your teen gets bright light exposure in the morning is one tip for keeping their body clock in check. This may be via sunlight or via artificial light on the blue light wave (e.g. fluoro lights).

Teen Sleep Tips – Summary

(a) Set a consistent bedtime during the school week. If possible, also set a weekend bedtime (no more than two hours later than their school-night bedtime).

(b) Provide a calm, quiet (homework-free) environment in the lead-up to bedtime. In the same way that you use a dimmer switch to create a tranquil and relaxing atmosphere at night, there should be a dimmer switch to turn down the stimulation in your home as the evening wears on.

(c) Avoid letting your teen have long 'catch-up' sleep-ins at the weekend, which can impact on their sleep pressure.

So that's it. We really hope we have been able to teach you to become your own sleep therapist and to help your child with their sleep problem.

Good night!

References

AAP Council On Communications And Media (2016). 'Media use in school-aged children and adolescents'. *Pediatrics*, 138, e20162592.

American Academy of Sleep Medicine (2014). *International Classification of Sleep Disorders* (3rd edition) (ICSD-3). Darien, Illinois, USA: American Academy of Sleep Medicine.

Bartel, K., & Gradisar, M. (2017). 'New directions in the link between technology use and sleep in young people'. In Sona Nevsimalova & Oliviero Bruni (eds.), *Sleep Disorders in Children*, pp. 69–80, Springer International Publishing, Switzerland.

Bartel, K., Gradisar, M., Williamson, P. (2015). 'Protective and risk factors for adolescent sleep: A meta-analytic review'. *Sleep Medicine Reviews*, 21, 72–85.

Bartel, K., Scheeren, R., & Gradisar, M. (2017). 'Altering adolescents' pre-bedtime phone use to achieve better sleep health'. *Health Communication*. In Press.

Bartel, K., Williamson, P., van Maanen, A., Cassoff, J., Meijer, A. M., Oort, F., & Gradisar, M. (2016). 'Protective and risk factors associated with adolescent sleep: Findings from Australia, Canada and The Netherlands'. *Sleep Medicine*, 26, 97–103.

Baum, K. T., Desai, A., Field, J., Miller, L. E., Rausch, J., Beebe, D. W. (2014). 'Sleep restriction worsens mood and emotion regulation in adolescents'. *Journal of Child Psychology & Psychiatry*, 55, 180–90.

Cain, N., & Gradisar, M. (2010). 'Electronic media use and sleep in school-aged children and adolescents: A review'. *Sleep Medicine*, 11, 735–42.

Cajochen, C. (2007). 'Alerting effects of light'. *Sleep Medicine Review*, 11, 453–64.

Carskadon, M. A. (2011). 'Sleep in adolescents: The perfect storm'. *Pediatric Clinics of North America*, 58, 637–47.

Carskadon, M. A., & Dement, W. C. (2005). 'Monitoring and staging human sleep'. In M. H. Kryger, T. Roth, W. C. Dement (eds.), *Principles and Practice of Sleep Medicine*, pp. 1359–77. Elsevier, Philadelphia, PA.

Carskadon, M. A., Harvey, K., Duke, P., Anders, T. F., Litt, I. F., & Dement, W. C. (1980). 'Pubertal changes in daytime sleepiness'. *Sleep*, 2, 453–60.

Crowley, S. J., & Carskadon, M. A. (2010). 'Modifications to weekend recovery sleep delay circadian phase in older adolescents'. *Chronobiology International*, 27, 1469–92.

Czeisler, C. A., Duffy, J. F., Shanahan, T. L., Brown, E. N., Mitchell, J. F., Rimmer, D. W., Ronda, J. M., Silva, E. J., Allan, J. S., Emens, J. S., Dijk, D., Kronauer, R. E. (1999). 'Stability, precision, and near-24-hour period of the human circadian pacemaker'. *Science,* 284, 2177–81.

Dahl, R. E., & Harvey, A. G. (2007). 'Sleep in children and adolescents with behavioral and emotional disorders'. *Sleep Medicine Clinics,* 2, 501–11.

Dewald, J. F., Short, M. A., Gradisar, M., Oort, F. J., Meijer, A. M. (2012). 'The Chronic Sleep Reduction Questionnaire (CSRQ): a cross-cultural comparison and validation in Dutch and Australian adolescents'. *Journal of Sleep Research,* 5, 584–94.

Drake, C., Richardson, G., Roehrs, T., Scofield, H., & Roth, T. (2004). 'Vulnerability to stress-related sleep disturbance and hyperarousal'. *Sleep,* 27, 285–91.

Evenson, K. R., Goto, M. M., & Furberg, R. D., (2015). 'Systematic review of the validity and reliability of consumer-wearable activity Trackers'. *International Journal of Behavioral Nutrition.* DOI 10.1186/s12966-015-0314-1

Ferber, R., (2006). *Solve Your Child's Sleep Problems* (2nd edition). New York, NY: Fireside.

Galland, B. C., Taylor, B. J., Elder, D. E., & Herbison, P. (2012). 'Normal sleep patterns in infants and children: A systematic review of observational studies'. *Sleep Medicine Reviews,* 16, 213–22.

Gangwisch, J. E., Babiss, L. A., Malaspina, D., Turner, J. B., Zammit, G. K., & Posner, K. (2010). 'Earlier parental set bedtimes as a protective factor against depression and suicidal ideation'. *Sleep*, 33, 97–106.

Gradisar, M., Dohnt, H., Gardner, G., Paine, S., Starkey, K., Menne, A., Slater, A., Wright, H., Hudson, J. L., Weaver, E., & Trenowden, S. (2011a). 'A randomized controlled trial of cognitive-behavior therapy plus bright light therapy for adolescent delayed sleep phase disorder'. *Sleep*, 34, 1671–80.

Gradisar, M., Gardner, G., & Dohnt, H. (2011b). 'Recent worldwide sleep patterns and problems during adolescence: A review and meta-analysis of age, region, and sleep'. *Sleep Medicine*, 12, 110–18.

Gradisar, M., & Short, M. (2013). 'Sleep hygiene and environment: Role of technology'. In A. R. Wolfson and H. Montgomery-Downs (eds.), *Oxford Handbook of Infant, Child, and Adolescent Sleep and Behaviour*, (pp. 113–26). New York, USA: Oxford University Press.

Gradisar, M., Wolfson, A. R., Harvey, A., Hale, L., Rosenberg, R., & Czeisler, C. A. (2013). 'The sleep and technology use of Americans: Findings from the 2011 National Sleep Foundation's "Sleep in America" Poll'. *Journal of Clinical Sleep Medicine*, 9, 1291–9.

Heath, M., Sutherland, C., Bartel, K., Gradisar, M., Williamson, P., Lovato, N., & Micic, G. (2014). 'Does one hour of bright or filtered short-wavelength tablet screen-light have a meaningful effect on adolescent's pre-bedtime alertness, sleep and daytime functioning?' *Chronobiology International*, 31, 496–505.

Hiller, R. M., Lovato, N., Gradisar, M., Oliver, M., & Slater, A. (2014). 'Trying to fall asleep while catastrophising: what sleep-disordered adolescents think and feel'. *Sleep Medicine*, 15, 96–103.

Iglowstein, I., Jenni, O. G., Molinari, L., Largo, R. H. (2003). 'Sleep duration from infancy to adolescence: Reference values and generational trends'. *Pediatrics*, 111, 302–7.

Jenni, O. G., Borbély, A. A., & Achermann, P. (2004). 'Development of the nocturnal sleep electroencephalogram in human infants'. *American Journal of Physiology: Regulatory, Integrative and Comparative Physiology*, 286, R528–38.

King, D., Gradisar, M., Drummond, A., Lovato, N., Wessel, J., Micic, G., Douglas, P., & Defabbro, P. (2013). 'The impact of violent videogaming on adolescent sleep-wake activity'. *Journal of Sleep Research*, 22, 137–43.

Kotagal, S. (2009). 'Parasomnias in childhood'. *Sleep Medicine Reviews*, 13, 157–68.

Krauchi, K., Cajochen, C., & Wirz-Justice, A. (1997). 'A relationship between heat loss and sleepiness: Effects of postural change and melatonin administration'. *Journal of Applied Physiology*, 83, 134–9.

Kryger, M. H., Roth, T., & Dement, W. C. (eds.), *Principles and Practice of Sleep Medicine* (5th edition, pp. 16–26). St Louis: Elsevier Saunders.

Lo, J. C., Ong, J. L., Leong, R. L. F., Gooley, J. J., & Chee, M. W. L. (2016). 'Cognitive performance, sleepiness, and mood in partially sleep deprived adolescents: The Need for Sleep Study'. *Sleep*, 39, 687–98.

Miller, C. B., Espie, C. A., Epstein, D. R., Friedman, L., Morin, C. M., Pigeon, W. R., Spielman, A. J., & Kyle, S. D. (2014). 'The evidence base of sleep restriction therapy for treating insomnia disorder'. *Sleep Medicine Reviews*, 18, 415–24.

Miller, W. R., & Rollnick, S. (2012). *Motivational interviewing: Helping people change* (3rd edition). New York: Guildford Press.

Mindell, J. A., Meltzer, L. J., Carskadon, M. A., & Chervin, R. D. 'Developmental aspects of sleep hygiene: Findings from the 2004 National Sleep Foundation "Sleep in America" Poll'. *Sleep Medicine*, 10, 771–9.

Moberly, N. J., & Watkins, E. R. (2008). 'Ruminative self-focus and negative affect: An experience sampling study'. *Journal of Abnormal Psychology*, 117, 314–23.

Muris, P., Murckelbach, H., Gadet, B., & Moulaert, V. (2000). 'Fears, worries and scary dreams in 4 to 12-year-old children: their content, developmental pattern, and origins'. *Journal of Clinical Child Psychology*, 29, 43–52.

National Sleep Foundation (2006). *2006 'Sleep in America' Poll: Summary of findings*. Washington, DC: National Sleep Foundation.

Olds, T., Maher, C., Blunden, S., Matricciani, L. (2010). 'Normative data on the sleep habits of Australian children and adolescents'. *Sleep*, 33, 1381–8.

Paine, S., & Gradisar, M. (2011). 'A randomised controlled trial of cognitive-behaviour therapy for behavioural insomnia of childhood in school-aged children'. *Behaviour Research and Therapy*, 49, 379–88.

Reynolds, C., Gradisar, M., Afrin, K., Perry, A., Wolfe, J., & Short, M. A. (2016). 'Adolescents who perceive fewer consequences of risk-taking choose to switch off games later at night'. *Acta Paediatrica*, 104, e222–e227.

Sadeh, K. (2005). 'Cognitive-behavioral treatment for childhood sleep disorders'. *Clinical Psychology Review*, 25, 612–28.

Short, M. A., Gradisar, M., Wright, H., Lack, L. C., Dohnt, H., & Carskadon, M. A. (2011). 'Time for bed: Parent-set bedtimes associated with improved sleep and daytime functioning in adolescents'. *Sleep*, 34, 797–800.

Short, M.A., & Louca, M. (2015). 'Sleep deprivation leads to mood deficits in healthy Adolescents'. *Sleep Medicine*, 16, 987–93.

Smith, L., Gradisar, M., King, D. L., & Short, M. A. (2017). 'Intrinsic and extrinsic predictors of video gaming behavior and adolescent bedtimes: The relationship between flow states, self-perceived risk-taking, device accessibility, parent-regulation of media and bedtime'. *Sleep Medicine*, 30, 64–70.

Smith, L., King, D.L., Richardson, C., Roane, B., & Gradisar, M. (2017). 'Mechanisms influencing older adolescents' bedtimes during videogaming: the roles of game difficulty and flow'. *Sleep Medicine*. In Press.

Spielman, A. J. (1986). 'Assessment of insomnia'. *Clinical Psychology Review*, 6, 11–25.

Taylor, D. J., Jenni, O. G., Acebo, C., & Carskadon, M. A. (2005). 'Sleep tendency during extended wakefulness: insights into adolescent sleep regulation and behavior'. *Journal of Sleep Research*, 14, 239–44.

Van der Lely, S., Frey, S., Garbazza, C., Wirz-Justice, A., Jenni, O. G., Steiner, R., Wolf, S., Cajochen, C., Bromundt, V., & Schmidt, C. (2015). 'Blue blocker glasses as a counter-measure for alerting effects of evening light-emitting diode screen exposure in male teenagers'. *Journal of Adolescent Health*, 56, 113–19.

Van Dongen, H. P. A., Maislin, G., Mullington, J. M., & Dinges, D. F. (2003). 'The cumulative cost of additional wakefulness: Dose-response effects on neurobehavioural functions and sleep physiology from chronic sleep restriction and total sleep deprivation'. *Sleep*, 26, 117–26.

Weaver, E., Gradisar, M., Dohnt, H., Lovato, N., & Douglas, P. (2010). 'The effect of pre-sleep video game playing on adolescent sleep'. *Journal of Clinical Sleep Medicine*, 6, 184–9.

Wolfe, J., Kar, K., Perry, A., Reynolds, C., Gradisar, M., & Short, M. A. (2014). 'Single night video game use leads to sleep loss and attention deficits in older adolescents'. *Journal of Adolescence*, 37, 1003–9.

Further Reading

Addressing general anxiety problems in children:

Cathy Creswell & Lucy Willetts (2018). *Helping Your Child with Fears and Worries* (2nd edition). Robinson.

Ronal Rapee, Ann Wignall, Susan H. Spence, Vanessa Cobham, Heidi Lyneham (2009). *Helping Your Anxious Child* (2nd edition). New Harbinger.

Appendix

Resources related to this book:

- Sleep-wake diary

- Weekly sleep schedule

- Quiet activities menu

- Helping your child to identify how emotions feel in their body

- Challenging worry thoughts

- Rating your emotions: Feeling thermometer

- Exposure steps and reward ladder

SLEEP DIARY

(introduced in Part II, chapter 4)

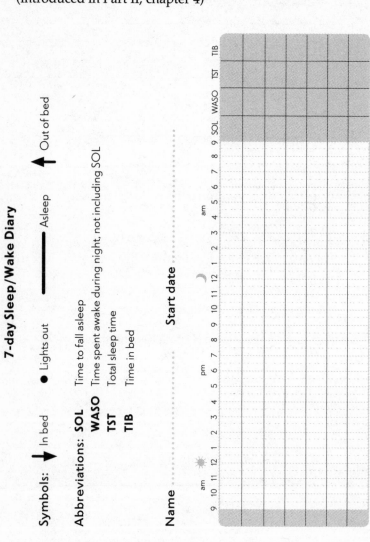

WEEKLY SLEEP SCHEDULE

For Bedtime Restriction or Sleep Restriction

	Quiet time	Bedtime	Wake-up time
Week 1 Date			
Week 2 Date			
Week 3 Date			

QUIET ACTIVITIES MENU

Pre-bedtime activities	Quiet ratings	Quiet menu	Times
List as many activities that your child can do between dinner time and sleep time	For each activity, give it a 'quiet rating' – with 1 being very quiet and relaxing and 10 being very stimulating	List all activities that you agree are 'quiet' activities	Write in your child's new bedtime. Then provide a timeframe for when the child can do each activity (between dinner and bedtime)

Where do you feel emotions in your body?

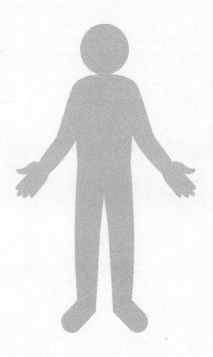

Challenging Worry Thoughts

Worry thought	How true?	Evidence for	Evidence against	How true now?	A balanced thought

Rating Your Emotions:
Feeling Thermometer

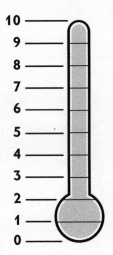

Exposure Ladder

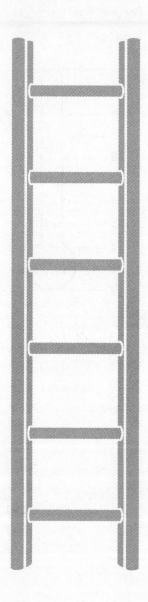

Acknowledgements

While we have provided some references to research articles in this book, the strategies we present also draw on work by many other researchers and clinicians in the child sleep and anxiety fields. The book is particularly influenced by the work of Leon Lack, Helen Wright, Cathy Creswell, Jennifer Hudson, Ron Rapee, Avi Sadeh and Mary Carskadon. We would also like to thank Polly Waite and Andrew McAleer, who provided invaluable feedback on the original drafts of this book. Many trainee and clinical psychologists, from the Child & Adolescent Sleep Clinic at Flinders University, have contributed to the research projects that form the foundations of the interventions presented in this book. Thank you to Sarah Paine, Erin Leahy, Sarah Watherston, Neralie Cain and Emma Hunt, who have led many of these projects, and the dozens of sleep therapists and admin people over the past decade. We would also like to thank our families for their patience and understanding of the writing process and the many early morning/late night cross-continent/time-zone Skyping. Rachel would like to particularly mention Simon, Oliver, Charlotte, Harrison and Alex. Michael would like to thank

Amy, Nathaniel, Ethan and Rossi. Last, but certainly not least, thank you to all of the families with whom we have worked, and who have also taught us, over the years.

Index

Note: page numbers in **bold** refer to diagrams and information contained in tables.